APPLICATION OF LASERS IN NEUROSURGERY

APPLICATION OF LASERS IN NEUROSURGERY

LEONARD J. CERULLO, M.D.
*Associate Professor of Surgery (Neurosurgery)
Northwestern University Medical School
Director, Chicago Neurosurgical Center
Chicago, Illinois*

YEAR BOOK MEDICAL PUBLISHERS, INC.
Chicago • London • Boca Raton

Copyright © 1988 by Year Book Medical Publishers, Inc. All rights reserved. No part of this publication may be reproduced, stored in a retrieval system, or transmitted, in any form or by any means—electronic, mechanical, photocopying, recording, or otherwise—without prior written permission from the publisher. Printed in the United States of America.

1 2 3 4 5 6 7 8 9 0 K R   92 91 90 89 88

Library of Congress Cataloging-in-Publication Data

Cerullo, L. J. (Leonard J.)
  Application of lasers in neurosurgery.

  Includes bibliographies and index.
  1. Nervous system—Surgery. 2. Lasers in surgery.
I. Title. [DNLM: 1. Laser Surgery. 2. Nervous
System—surgery. WL 368 C418a]
RD593.C38   1988   617'.48   87-21065
ISBN 0-8151-1509-1

Sponsoring Editor: Daniel J. Doody
Assistant Director, Manuscript Services: Frances M. Perveiler
Production Project Managers: Robert Allen Reedtz/Etta Worthington
Proofroom Supervisor: Shirley E. Taylor

This book is dedicated to the founding members of the Laser Association of Neurological Surgeons International, to those who lit the light and kept it burning

Contributors

Robert E. Anderson, B.S.
Assistant Professor of Neurosurgery, Mayo Medical School, Mayo Foundation, Rochester, Minnesota

Julian E. Bailes, M.D.
Clinical Instructor, Division of Neurosurgery, Department of Surgery, Northwestern University Medical School
Chicago, Illinois

J. Thomas Brown, M.D.
Assistant Professor of Surgery (Neurosurgery), Northwestern University Medical School; Attending Physician, Northwestern Memorial Hospital, Chicago Neurosurgical Center, Chicago, Illinois

Leonard J. Cerullo, M.D.
Associate Professor of Surgery (Neurosurgery), Northwestern University Medical School, Director, Chicago Neurosurgical Center, Chicago, Illinois

W. Craig Clark, M.D., Ph.D.
Assistant Professor, Department of Neurosurgery, University of Tennessee, Memphis, Tennessee

Max Epstein, Ph.D.
Professor of Electrical and Biomedical Engineering, Northwestern University, Evanston, Illinois

Patrick J. Kelly, M.D.
Professor of Neurosurgery, Mayo Clinic and Mayo Medical School; St. Mary's Hospital and Rochester Methodist Hospital, Rochester, Minnesota

Edward R. Laws, Jr., M.D.
Chairman, Department of Neurosurgery, George Washington University School of Medicine, Washington, D.C.

Carolyn J. Mackety, R.N.
Senior Vice President, Laser Centers of America, Cincinnati, Ohio

David G. McLone, M.D., Ph.D.
Professor of Surgery (Neurosurgery), Northwestern University Medical School; Head, Division of Pediatric Neurosurgery, Children's Memorial Hospital, Chicago, Illinois

Charles R. Neblett, M.D.
Clinical Assistant Professor, Department of Neurosurgery, Baylor College of Medicine; Active Staff, Methodist Hospital; Board of Trustees, The Diagnostic Center Hospital, Houston, Texas

Thomas G. Polanyi, Ph.D.
Adjunct Professor of Otolaryngology, Boston University School of Medicine, Boston, Massachusetts; Chief Scientist, Cooper Lasersonics, Hospital Division, Marlboro, Massachusetts

Stephen K. Powers, M.D.
Assistant Professor and Acting Chief, Division of Neurosurgery, University of North Carolina; North Carolina Memorial Hospital, Chapel Hill, North Carolina

Matthew R. Quigley, M.D.
West Pennsylvania Hospital, Pittsburgh, Pennsylvania

Jon H. Robertson, M.D.
Associate Professor, Department of Neurosurgery, University of Tennessee; Baptist Memorial Hospital and William F. Bowld Hospital, Memphis, Tennessee

Tod B. Sloan, M.D., Ph.D.
Assistant Professor, Northwestern University; Director, Neurosurgical Anesthesia, Director, Neurophysiologic Monitoring, Northwestern Memorial Hospital, Chicago, Illinois

Marion L. Walker, M.D.
Associate Professor of Pediatrics, Associate Professor of Surgery (Neurosurgery), University of Utah Medical Center; Chairman, Division of Pediatric Neurosurgery, Primary Children's Medical Center, Salt Lake City, Utah

Robert E. Wharen, Jr., M.D.
Instructor of Neurosurgery, Mayo Medical School, Mayo Clinic—Jacksonville, Jacksonville, Florida

Preface

It is difficult to justify any technologic tool in surgery by quantifying results. If the instrument appears to have inherent value, a prospective study is morally difficult to design. There is no question, for instance, that the bipolar cautery is an invaluable addition to the neurosurgical armamentarium. On the other hand, there are few articles showing statistical validity to the superiority of the bipolar over monopolar coagulating methods. It is even more difficult to justify improvements on the theme, such as the "nonstick" bipolar. On the other hand, few would deny the major improvement that "nonstick" bipolar cautery has afforded both surgeon and patient. For these technologic advances, then, we are forced to borrow the legal term, "res ipse loquitor," the thing speaks for itself.

Few neurosurgeons who have had the opportunity to use laser in an appropriate fashion would deny the inherent value of the precision and gentleness afforded by this instrument. Accordingly, the use of laser has burgeoned in neurosurgery. Congresses, workshops, and other educational forums have been designed to instruct the neurosurgical community in laser from physics through application. Meanwhile, residency programs have incorporated laser training into their conventional educational program. Lasers, like microscopes and bipolars, have become an accepted part of the neurosurgeon's armamentarium.

This book, dedicated to the founding members of the Laser Association of Neurological Surgeons International, is designed to offer the practicing or training neurosurgeon fundamental information regarding laser physics, safety, application, and direction. The uses of laser are not limited, nor are the wavelengths limited, to those discussed in this brief treatise. On the other hand, it is hoped that this book will pique the imagination of the reader to develop further, to investigate further, and to capitalize further on the use of light energy in surgery.

The future of laser neurosurgery is limited only by the imagination of the surgeons.

LEONARD J. CERULLO, M.D.

Contents

Preface   ix

1/ **Prologue** *by Thomas G. Polanyi*   **1**

2/ **Power: From Instrument to Tissue** *by Max Epstein*   **10**

3/ **Laser Safety** *by Carolyn J. Mackety*   **27**

4/ **Anesthesiologic Considerations** *by Tod B. Sloan*   **40**

5/ **Extra-axial Tumor Removal** *by Leonard J. Cerullo*   **49**

6/ **Pediatric Neurosurgery** *by Marion L. Walker and David G. McLone*   **60**

7/ **Glial Neoplasms: Conventional and Stereotactic Applications** *by Patrick J. Kelly*   **82**

8/ **Intraspinal Tumors** *by Jon H. Robertson and W. Craig Clark*   **100**

9/ **Vascular Applications: The Thermal Scale** *by Charles R. Neblett*   **110**

10/ **Neuroablative Procedures** *by J. Thomas Brown*   **115**

11/ **Theoretical Neurosurgery** *by Matthew R. Quigley and Julian E. Bailes*   **129**

12/ **Photochemotherapy** *by Stephen K. Powers*   **137**

13/ **Photoradiation Therapy of Malignant Brain Tumors** *by Robert E. Wharen, Jr., Robert E. Anderson, and Edward R. Laws, Jr.*   **156**

Index   173

1 Prologue

THOMAS G. POLANYI, PH.D.

I am honored and delighted that Dr. Cerullo has asked me, a physicist, to write a prologue to this book. I am delighted because, twenty years after the discovery of the potential surgical utility of carbon dioxide (CO_2) lasers — an event that I witnessed in my laboratory and that has deeply affected my professional career ever since — the benefits to patients of this and other lasers are continuing to expand.

The role of lasers in the complex tasks of neurosurgery is still evolving. This becomes clear when reading the contributions to this book of the pioneering surgeons in this field. It also becomes clear that this role will become established through new ideas, new approaches, novel instrumentation, and much hard and dedicated work.

In what follows, I will attempt to evoke how lasers were introduced to operative (nonophthalmic) surgery, how cherished initial hopes had to be abandoned, and how slowly accumulating experiences in the field of laryngeal microsurgery benefited other fields, neurosurgery in particular.

The successful realization of the first laser — the ruby laser — by Maiman in 1960 created enormous excitement in the scientific world, including the medical world.

The pioneering work of G. Meyer-Schwickerath in the early 1950s sensitized opthalmologists to the use of light sources in producing therapeutic lesions in the retina. They were the first, in 1961, to experiment with this laser in surgery. Soon the advantage for retinal surgery of this new light source was established, and by 1964 hundreds of patients had been treated. Since that time the use of lasers in ophthalmology has continuously expanded. Currently, the practice of ophthalmology without lasers is inconceivable, and ophthalmologists are still the largest medical users of lasers.

Surgeons in other fields, including neurosurgeons, were also fascinated by the laser. One hope was that irradiating cancers with laser light would lead to more effective cancer therapy. However, these hopes were quickly dashed by the experimental work that followed. There was no reason then, nor is there any today, for this belief. Nevertheless, as later developments have shown, lasers have found a significant role in the treatment of selected cancers, albeit in an entirely different usage. Indeed, it can be anticipated confidently that the association of lasers with the ever-advancing methods of intraoperative real-time diagnosis will lead to a further expansion of laser use in cancer surgery. But this is the future.

The early history of the use of ruby and neodymium (Nd)-in-glass lasers in neurosurgery, which ended in 1967, was summarized in 1974 by Stellar et al., who participated in this early work and who later pioneered the introduction of the CO_2 laser into neurosurgery:

When ruby laser pulses of a few joules were first applied to tissues, it was found that no effect occurred unless the radiation was focused to a small spot. If a focused spot of either ruby or neodymium lasers was used, small volumes of tissue of about 1 mm were damaged by conversion of the radiation into heat. Small vessels less than 0.5 mm in diameter in the path of the beam were coagulated, while larger ones would be ruptured with obviously potentially disastrous consequences, e.g., in the brain. . . . High-energy pulses focused on tissues created more violent tissue destruction with ejection of disrupted material in the form of a plume created by sudden steam formation. At still higher energies and using larger focal spots, 1/2 to 1 cm, veritable shock waves were created that in experimental animals led to rapid fatalities. . . .

It soon became apparent that to destroy cancers, high-energy pulses focused to a small spot of 1 sq mm had to be used and that each impact made little impression on a neoplastic mass just a few centimeters in diameter. Hundreds of impacts, even thousands, are necessary to destroy such a mass completely, a thing necessary for cure. . . . In addition, it was found that at the required energy levels viable cancer cells could be disseminated by the pulse and/or the shock wave with obvious severe danger of internal transplantation. These various effects have been studied and reported by several authors. Stellar, Fox et al. and Lampert describe experiments in which brain tissue of animals such as mice, cats, and dogs has been driven into cranial openings by ruby laser pulses, hemorrhages have occurred, and the impacts have been followed by immediate death or severe neurological damage. . . .

Transillumination of the tumor by the red beam of the ruby laser of 0.69 μm was thought to alter the enzyme systems of the neoplastic cells with the result that their metabolic processes were reversed and the cells died and were resorbed . . . Regression did not occur in our own series of transplantable ependymoblastomas and melanomas in mice similarly treated with the ruby laser. Some of these were cured, but only if the tumor was small and visibly destroyed by large numbers of laser impacts. . . .

It became obvious that pulsed ruby and neodymium lasers as used were not suitable tools either for cancer therapy or for operative surgery.[1]

The discouragement concerning the use of lasers in operative surgery was caused by the characteristics of the lasers available to these early workers, the ruby and the Nd-in-glass. Electromagnetic energy at the wavelength of these lasers, 0.69 and 1.06 μm, respectively, is poorly absorbed by biologic tissues. In addition, these lasers operate only in short pulses. The discouragement with lasers for surgery lasted a long time, continuing into the period when more suitable lasers had been discovered, particularly the CO_2 laser discovered by Patel in 1964. By 1965, various means had been found to increase the power output of this laser, which operated in the continuous mode at 10.6 μm to the unprecedented level of hundreds of watts.

At that time, I was directing the gas laser research and development work of Laser Inc., a subsidiary of the American Optical Corporation. Early in 1966, Dr. William Z. Yahr called me asking whether he could do an experiment with the CO_2 laser I had operating in the laboratory. Dr. Yahr was then a fourth-year surgical resident at Montefiore Hospital in New York. He had been trying for some time to perfect a nonocclusive side-to-end vessel anastomosis and was searching for an optimal means to create the passage between the common walls of efferent and afferent vessels joined by a glue. He thought that he might use a laser for this purpose. He tried this repeatedly with an Nd-in-glass laser in another facility of the American Optical Corporation in Southbridge, Mass., where this laser had been discovered. He had encountered difficulties in this work and he realized that these were caused by the lack of absorption by tissues of the energy of the Nd laser. He thought that by staining the tissues with copper sulfate he would overcome the problems. However, a new problem presented itself at the power and energy levels necessary to create the desired passage: the glued common wall was disrupted by the impact of the beam. With the help of physicists at Southbridge, Dr. Yahr explored the absorption characteristics of biologic tissues and concluded: "Briefly, tissues are almost perfect black bodies for the molecular nitrogen–carbon dioxide laser and relatively good black bodies for the argon ion laser." This was the background to Dr. Yahr's call to me.

Our CO_2 laser was a typical physics laboratory laser; in particular, the focused beam was stationary. After preliminary trials, Dr. Yahr brought anesthetized dogs to the laboratory, and soon numerous surgical operations were performed by slowly moving the anesthetized animal under the fixed focused beam. With growing enthusiasm, Dr. Yahr and his senior colleague Dr. J. K. Strully used the focused CO_2 laser beam to make skin incisions, cut through muscle and fascia, perform laparotomies, and resect liver lobes. It seemed miraculous to see that not only did tissues part, as if by a steel scalpel, by invisible "immaterial" energy, but tissue bleeding was minimal. These were my first contacts with the surgical world and the first operations at which I had ever assisted. When the liver resection was made, I thought that there was much bleeding, and I must confess that my "inner man" was not quite well for 24 hours. I was assured, however, that the bleeding I had seen was nothing compared with the same operation performed with a steel scalpel.

The enthusiasm of Yahr and Strully for this new potential surgical instrument was obvious and infectious. It led to the development of the first CO_2 laser system for surgery. This was a self-contained, movable system with beam delivery through a hand-held focusing system, later named the focusing hand piece, attached to the distal end of an articulated arm. The point of impact of the movable beam was marked by a set of white light cross hairs. It became available for surgical research in spring of 1967. In an article that appeared at the end of 1966, Yahr and Strully wrote:

> Using a nitrogen carbon-dioxide laser . . . clean, dry skin incisions which heal as well or better than scalpel controls were fashioned. Bone, liver, kidney, and lung can be cleanly divided. . . . The future medical applications of laser energy are many. Leaving

the realm of arterial surgery one may consider some of the following uses. . . . Many brain tumors, and some congenital defects, block the reflow of cerebrospinal fluid. . . . A flexible bundle carrying both sight and laser could be introduced into one of the cavities . . . and a simple decompression . . . operation performed as an initial step in the patient's treatment. . . . laser beams delivered through flexible bundles could be employed [to] fracture stones blocking important biologic duct systems. . . . It appears probable that the nitrogen carbon-dioxide laser will find a place to make rapid skin incisions, divide certain organs without blood loss, and to anastomose vessels as an adjunct to standard techniques.[2]

In March 1967, American Optical's CO_2 laser system for surgery with an articulated arm was exhibited at the meeting of the American College of Surgeons in New York City. The news spread rapidly; already in 1967, Dr. R. Edlich, in the laboratory of Prof. O. H. Wangensteen at the University of Minnesota, Minneapolis, showed that with the unfocused beam of the CO_2 laser the parietal cells could be devitalized without damage to the lamina muscularis mucosae. In the same laboratory, Drs. R. Gounzalez and R. L. Goodale used the defocused beam to obtain hemostasis of subcapsular superficial lesions of the liver and of deep gastric erosions. They found that hemostasis was obtained much more rapidly than with electrocoagulation.

Many other short- and long-range investigations were soon started. Apart from Dr. Edlich's investigation, which might be described loosely as functional surgery, the majority of these investigations were motivated by the ancient and recurring dream of bloodless surgery. One of these investigations indirectly had an important bearing on the introduction of the CO_2 laser to neurosurgery. This was the extensive investigation on burn débridement started in 1968 by Dr. James Fidler, who was associated with the laser laboratory of Dr. Leon Goldman and the Shriner's Burn Institute of the University of Cincinnati. Dr. Fidler reported his initial results at the Gordon Research Conference on Lasers in Medicine and Surgery in summer 1968. Participating in the conference was Dr. Stanley Stellar. He recognized the profound differences between the effect of this laser beam on tissues and those of the ruby and Nd-in-glass lasers with which he had worked until then. Immediately following the conference, he came to our laboratory and performed a variety of surgical experiments on cat scalp, dura, brain, and spinal cord. He was extremely encouraged, and this was the start of his extensive, classic experimental investigations on the use of the CO_2 laser in neurosurgery, first at St Barnabas Hospital in Bronx, N.Y., and later at St Barnabas Hospital in Livingston, N.J.

In the first article on this subject in 1970, we wrote:

The ability of the CO_2 laser beam to cut tissue effectively was readily apparent from the outset and virtually all tissues yielded to it without difficulty. Haemostasis was excellent in cats, rabbits and mice. . . .

Tumours could be made to disappear by vaporization directly to a gas or they could be incised in the same manner as ordinary tissue. . . .

To see a cancer disappear in smoke within a matter of a few minutes is remarkable. . . .
Minimal lesions of a predetermined size could be made quite easily, suggesting that functional neurosurgical procedures might well be developed with this new technique. . . .
Spinal cord pathways such as those subserving pain can also be easily destroyed, whenever they can be reached surgically. Whether the laser will compete effectively with current cryosurgical or radio-frequency methods cannot be predicted at present. . . .
Haemostasis with the CO_2 laser is good in all tissues since capillaries, veins and small arteries are readily coagulated if the power output is a few watts or more using a focused beam. Larger vessels will be perforated with resultant bleeding but experiments are now in progress in our laboratory to determine which parameters, particularly high intensity and defocusing, will prevent perforation of vessels before coagulating them. . . .
Computer control, with automatic scanning resulting from a suitable feed-back mechanism, might reduce the operating time for large tumours provided the neurosurgeon over-rides the instrument whenever necessary.[3]

With light and electron microscopic histologic studies, we showed the characteristics and the limited range of the tissue damage produced with the CO_2 laser. We summarized the advantages of the laser as follows:

(1) Ability to deliver a high intensity, directed, easily controllable beam of energy for the rapid and effective cutting, drilling or vaporization of tissue. (2) The lack of forced impact and, hence, gentleness of action on surrounding tissue. (3) A restriction of action when properly controlled to a distance of less than 1 mm from the edge of the beam. (4) The ability to destroy micro-organisms and to sterilize tissues during its application.[3]

In 1969, Dr. Stellar performed his first operation on a human. This was the first neurosurgical operation with a CO_2 laser and the first clinical use of the CO_2 laser on man. In the same 1970 article, we wrote:

One human brain tumour, a primary malignant glioblastoma multiforme, was treated surgically by means of the carbon dioxide laser on 26 May 1969. Previous conventional surgery and radiotherapy had already failed to help. This case showed the technical feasibility of using this laser in patients, since the neoplastic tissue was readily vaporized with no visible impact or other harmful effect on the surrounding brain. The clinical recovery from the operation during the early post-operative period was unusually good with lessening of the pre-existing neurological abnormalities. No attempt was made, because of the unfavourable location of the tumour in the dominant motor and speech area, to perform a radical destruction of neoplasm. Application of this method to the treatment of additional otherwise hopeless human brain tumours is now warranted.[3]

The way for further studies and clinical applications of the CO_2 laser in neurosurgery appeared to have been opened. But the use of this laser in neurosurgery remained dormant for many years.

As mentioned earlier, most of the initial investigations in surgery were based on the hoped-for hemostatic properties of the CO_2 laser. This search continued for most of the 1970s, even in the face of experimental evidence that the hemostatic properties of this laser were limited. The real surgical utility of the CO_2 laser emerged slowly from the work of Dr. Geza J. Jako, an otolaryngologist, which started in 1968. This led to combining the CO_2 laser beam with an operating microscope and to controlling the position of the focal spot in the visual field of the microscope by means of a micromanipulator. The first laryngeal operation with this instrumentation was performed in 1971 by Drs. M. Stuart Strong and Geza Jako of the Boston University Medical School. Recognition of the advantages of this new surgical modality for numerous operations in the aerodigestive tract spread rapidly, and soon it became the method of choice in many hands. Today, the CO_2 laser–operating microscope combination is universally recognized as an essential adjunct in laryneal microsurgery.

What makes the CO_2 laser modality so valuable in surgery of the aerodigestive tract are the following characteristics: (1) precise removal of tissues from a distance; (2) the ability to remove minimal tissue volumes with minimal adjacent tissue damage; (3) the ability to operate in restricted areas, and by the use of mirrors in areas not accessible to direct vision; (4) the lack of encumbrance by solid instruments of the restricted visual space available when operating in deep cavities; (5) lack of bleeding from capillaries and small vessels, which preserves the improved tissue diagnosis capability of the operating microscope; (6) the generally benign tissue reaction and uneventful healing of laser wounds.

I firmly believe that the more one or more of these characteristics are vital in an operation, the greater is the potential applicability of the CO_2 laser as a primary or adjunctive surgical modality. Gynecologic microsurgery, today one of the more extensive applications of CO_2 lasers in surgery, is based on these characteristics. It was inspired directly by the larnygeal work; indeed, the first gynecologic operations in 1974 took place in the operating rooms of laryngeal surgeons.

Investigation of the applicability of the CO_2 laser to neurosurgery was taken up in summer 1975 by Dr. Peter W. Ascher and his chief, Dr. F. Heppner, at the University Hospital in Graz, Austria. Building on the work of Stellar and encouraged by the expanding clinical applications of lasers, extensive animal experimentation was undertaken. Histologic studies with light, transmission, and scanning electron microscopy revealed a wealth of new information on tissue damage following application of laser energy, particularly to neural structures. On June 28, 1976, the first brain glioma operation was successfully performed in Graz. This was followed by an additional 69 operations in the short span of 9 months; at which time Dr. Ascher submitted for publication his monograph, *Der CO2-Laser in der Neurochirurgie*. The operations included treatment of 16 glioblastomas, 16 meningiomas, and other brain tumors, functional surgery, and spinal cord and peripheral nerve operations. In analyzing this work, Dr. Ascher pointed out the ability of directing the laser beam at any angle with mirrors, the noncontact action of the laser beam, and the avoidance of electrical stimulation of nervous tissue. He found the laser essential in removing firm central tumors. He also found that, in selected cases, shortened operating time and decreased postoperative morbidity may add up to an essential advantage. He foresees that, with the help of lasers, selected operations hitherto considered "major brain surgery" may become more routine. All but three of these operations were done "freehand." He noted that in the macroscopic approach, laser and conventional techniques have many similarities but that laser neuromicrosurgery with the micromanipulator is entirely new territory.

The operative momentum in Graz has continued. By 1985, 889 operations had been performed with lasers, 743 with the CO_2 laser and 146 with the Nd:YAG laser, discussed below. From these a wealth of experience, indications, contraindications, and partial indications have emerged.

Starting in 1977, Drs. Ascher and Heppner forcefully advocated the selective use of lasers in neurosurgery in numerous articles and lectures. This activity, and the support of Laser Industries, Ltd., Tel-Aviv, Israel, whose CO_2 laser instruments Drs. Ascher and Heppner used, stimulated the interest of many neurosurgeons in Europe, the Far East where efforts to apply the laser to neurosurgery had already been started, and the United States. In 1979, Prof. Aldo Fasano, a neurosurgeon, organized the first National Congress of the Italian Society for Laser Surgery in Torino, Italy. There a full session was devoted to the use of lasers in neurosurgery.

In the United States, neurosurgeons at different centers undertook basic experimenal and clinical investigations. Seminars and teaching courses were instituted. Dr. Leonard Cerullo established such a center of studies at Northwestern University Medical School in Chicago. Through his initiative, the first American Congress of Laser Neurosurgery was convened in October 1981. The three-day sessions were attended by over 100 neurosurgeons, and 20 papers were presented and discussed. Two more such conferences were held in Chicago in the following two years with increasing participation. Basic investigations, analysis, and exploration of the applications of lasers to neurosurgery had acquired the needed momentum.

During the time these developments were taking place, lasers other than the CO_2 laser started to play a significant role in neurosurgery. The most important of these for neurosurgery is the Nd:YAG laser. The output of this laser is continuous, contrary to the pulsed characteristics of the Nd-in-glass found so unsuitable for surgery in the early 1960s. Radiation of this laser at 1.06 μm penetrates deeply into tissues, millimeters as opposed to microns for the CO_2 laser. For this reason its hemostatic properties are excellent. The first use of this laser in medicine became a reality through the untiring efforts, started in 1975, of Dr. Peter Kiefhaber and Dr. Gunther Nath, a physicist. Dr. Nath developed the first fiber capable of transmitting high-power Nd:YAG radiation. Introducing this fiber in one channel of a gastroscope, Dr. Kiefhaber developed methods for the endoscopic coagulation of massive gastrointestinal hemorrhages. These obtained clinical success in 1977 and stimulated much additional work with this laser. The Nd:YAG laser used in this work was developed by Messerschmitt-Bolkow-Blohm Medizintechnik of Munich. Many investigations related to the use of the Nd:YAG in medicine were undertaken there owing to the support of the Gesellschaft fuer Strahlenforschung, a semiofficial institute for the study of laser radiation. There, Dr. K. K. Jain pioneered the work on sutureless microvascular anastomosis with the Nd:YAG laser.

Prof. Oskar J. Beck pioneered the use of the Nd:YAG laser in neurosurgery starting in 1976. By July 1979, the Nd:YAG laser had been used in 103 neurosurgical operations in the Neurological Clinic of the University of Munich, 51 of these on meningiomas.

The radiation of the Nd:YAG, owing to its deep penetration into tissues, cannot be used for dissection in proximity to sensitive functioning tissue, but other characteristics of this radiation are important in neurosurgical applications. In addition to hemostasis as already mentioned, it can be used for coagulating sizable volumes; also, this radiation is transmitted through cerebrospinal fluid with little attenuation. Flexible fibers are routinely available today that permit the development of very light hand-held accessories; endoscopic operations, as already undertaken by Dr. Ascher, are possible.

For many years, not surprisingly, a rivalry developed between proponents of the CO_2 and the Nd:YAG lasers. Today it behooves us to consider these lasers as complementary adjuncts to selected areas of surgery. Fasano has started using them in this way. Others select one or the other. Many of the early pioneers of surgery with lasers dreamed of the time when multiple-wavelength lasers would become available. Cooper LaserSonics now produces a surgical system delivering CO_2 and Nd:YAG laser radiations to explore areas of complementarity.

Through the work of Drs. J. Boggan, M. S. B. Edwards, and A. Fasano, the argon ion laser has also found specialized applications in neurosurgery, for example, to small arteriovenous malformations and in functional surgery. Earlier, this laser had been used only sporadically in experimental neurosurgery, by Dr. J. L. Fox for brain-tissue incision and by Dr. G. Maira for experimental aneurysm treatment.

The path to using lasers in neurosurgery has been tortuous. Expectations had to be modified and reduced, experience accumulated, approaches tried and discarded, new instrumentation developed, and many types of lasers tested. This work is continuing. No one surgical instrument or technique, or diagnostic method, is going to solve all the complex problems daily facing the surgeon. But all together, coordinated by the judgment and the skill of the surgeon, they will increasingly benefit patients, as discussed in the chapters of this book.

REFERENCES
1. Stellar S, Polanyi TG, Bredemeier HC: in Wolbarsht ML (ed): *Laser Applications in Medicine and Biology.* New York, Plenum Publishing Corp, 1974, vol 2, pp 250–252.
2. Yahr WZ, Strully JK: *J Assoc Adv Med Instr* 1966; 1:28–31.
3. Stellar S, Polanyi TG, Bredemeier HC: *Med Biol Eng* 1970; 549–558.

2 Power: From Instrument to Tissue
MAX EPSTEIN, PH.D.

The word *laser* is an acronym for light amplification by stimulated emission of radiation. Similar to all other light sources, laser energy is also in the form of electromagnetic radiation; however, it differs from conventional light in several major aspects. A conventional light source produces electromagnetic radiation over a large spectrum of frequencies or wavelengths, whereas laser energy consists of an electromagnetic wave of a single or extremely narrow range of wavelengths; i.e., it is monochromatic. Electromagnetic radiation from a conventional source is in the form of very short bursts that are uncorrelated with each other. On the other hand, laser radiation consists of a wave that continues to propagate over long periods and for a long distance, resulting in large coherence in time or length, respectively. Moreover, the wave front of the electromagnetic radiation of laser energy is uniform, leading to the property of spatial coherence. This latter property accounts for the ability to focus laser radiation to a very small spot and, consequently, to a very high energy density. It is this feature of concentrating laser light to a very small spot that makes it such an attractive tool in surgery, particularly in neurosurgery.

Electromagnetic radiation is absorbed or is emitted when a charged particle changes its energy state. In an atom, this occurs when an electron rises to a higher or drops to a lower energy state, respectively (Fig 2–1). Energy transitions in molecular systems can also cause absorption or emission of radiation. However, molecular transitions, which are associated with rotational and vibrational modes, have energies less than those in atomic systems. Consequently, electromagnetic radiation produced by atomic transitions are in the ultraviolet and visible range of the spectrum, whereas the molecular ones are usually in the infrared.

All spontaneous transitions occur randomly, resulting in the emission of electromagnetic radiation wherein its various segments, in time and space, remain uncorrelated. On the other hand, there are transitions, from a higher to a lower state, that are stimulated by photons of the electromagnetic radiation. These transitions emit additional photons of exactly the same wavelength, phase, and direction as the photons that stimulated the emission (Fig 2–2). To effect such stimulated transitions, the lasing medium must consist of excited atomic or molecular states; i.e., in atoms the electrons must reside in higher than usual energy states, or in molecules higher energy levels must be achieved by vibrational and rotational motions. Since under normal conditions higher energy states are less populated than lower ones, the population of energy states must be "inverted." Population inversion is therefore a prerequisite of lasing. To obtain a population inversion, the medium must be energized or "pumped." Pumping can be obtained by supplying energy to the lasing medium. Such energy can be

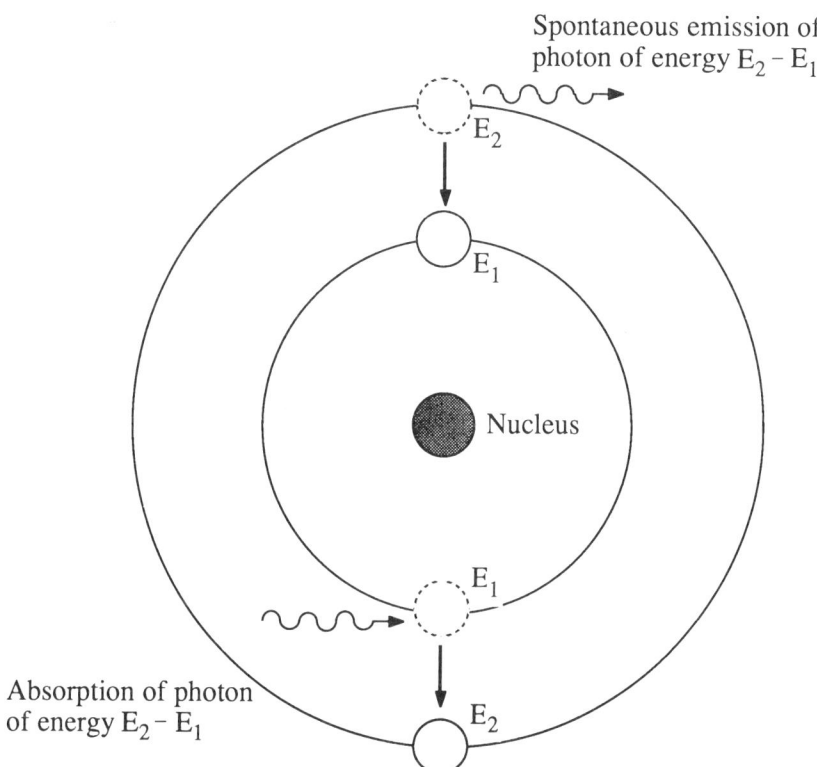

FIG 2–1.
Emission and absorption of electromagnetic radiation in an atom.

obtained by various means, including electric current, optical excitation, or chemical reactions.

Laser light is generated when stimulated emission exceeds the losses due to the absorption of the light in the medium. Thus, as the photons produced by stimulated emission proceed to multiply along a particular direction, a laser beam is generated. To allow for stimulated emission to render light beams of useful magnitude, the length of the beam path must be sufficiently long. A practical means of extending the length of the lasing medium is to place two opposing mirrors that reflect the beam back and forth between them. Such a structure forms a resonant cavity with one of the mirrors being partially transmitting to allow for the escape of the light beam (Fig 2–3).

Most lasers produce continuous radiation. However, when a shutter is placed inside the cavity, the population inversion can be built up to higher levels, and by removing the obstacle, the lasing energy can be obtained in a very short time,

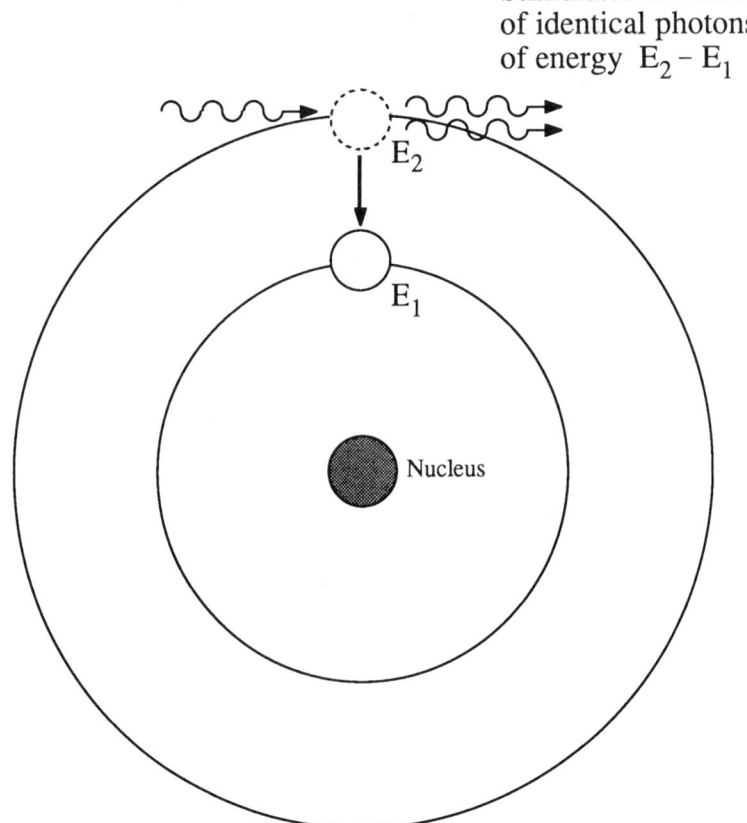

FIG 2–2.
Stimulated emission of electromagnetic radiation in an atom.

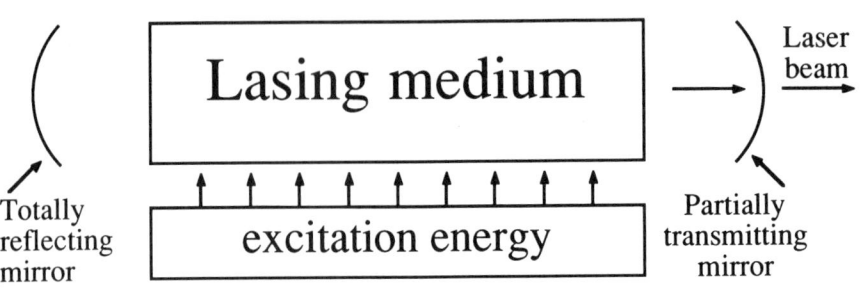

FIG 2–3.
Basic components of laser: lasing medium, pumping source, and optical cavity.

on the order of a few nanoseconds (nsec; billionth of a second). This mode of operation of the laser is referred to as "Q-switching" and derives its term from resonant systems of high Q (Q is the ratio of stored to dissipative energy in a resonant system).

In some lasers the stimulated emission can produce electromagnetic radiation at more than one wavelength or frequency simultaneously. If the different frequency modes are synchronized, i.e., their phases are in a fixed relationship or are locked together, high-power pulses are generated at the beat frequencies. Lasers operating in such manner are known as "mode-locked." Mode-locked lasers produce light energy in the form of very short pulses, shorter than Q-switched lasers, on the order of picoseconds (a millionth of a millionth of a second). In some cases mode-locking can occur inadvertently, as in the case of the argon-ion laser, which is used extensively in ophthalmology. Hence, when using such a laser in a continuous manner, special care must be taken to prevent sudden surges of high peak power by the generation of a mode-locked pulse output. Single-mode operation can be secured by placing a piece of transparent material with parallel faces (etalon) inside the laser cavity.

The structure of the laser cavity may contribute to the generation of laser beams of various geometries. These geometries are different patterns of the electromagnetic waves across the beam and, in analogy to microwave techniques, are referred to as spatial modes. The most natural and desirable pattern of the laser beam cross section is the form of a gaussian curve with the maximum at the center of the beam (Fig 2–4).

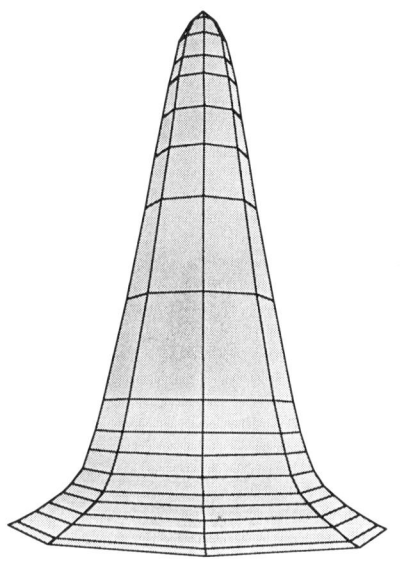

FIG 2–4.
Gaussian intensity distribution of a laser beam.

TYPES OF LASERS

The type of laser is defined by the lasing medium, which may consist of a gas, a liquid, or a solid. The lasing medium also determines the wavelength of the emitted light, with consequently different absorption of its energy in various body tissues. The first laser was constructed by T. H. Maiman in 1960. It utilizes a synthetic ruby crystal with chromium impurity, which is excited by a flashlamp. Since it renders light energy in very short pulses, its early applications in medicine were not successful, and it was eventually replaced by other lasers operating mostly in a continuous mode. The three types of lasers used most extensively in medical applications are the argon-ion laser, which emits in the blue-green range of the light spectrum, neodymium (Nd):YAG laser, which emits in the near-infrared at a wavelength of 1.06 μm, and carbon dioxide (CO_2) lasers, which radiate at 10.6 μm. Other lasers that find increasing use in medicine are the excimer (meaning excited dimer), dye, and, more recently, hydrogen fluoride (HF) or erbium-doped systems. A new laser, known as the free-electron laser (FEL), is currently being considered for medical research.

ARGON-ION LASER

The lasing medium of an argon-ion laser consists of an argon gas in a sealed tube that is excited by a high-voltage direct-current supply. Its efficiency is very low, below 0.1%, and, consequently it requires water cooling. It puts out light energy at several wavelengths, with the prevalent ones at 488 and 514.5 nm. Its output is continuous, although it can be pulsed in a mode-locked process. (As mentioned earlier, mode-locking may occur unintentionally, as may happen in the case of an argon-ion laser, which can produce dangerously high peak-power pulses. This can be prevented by placing in the laser cavity appropriate filtering devices that allow lasing at only one wavelength.) Light at wavelengths produced by the argon-ion laser passes unattenuated through clear media and is absorbed in red structures such as hemoglobin. Hence, argon-ion lasers have been used extensively in ophthalmology for the photocoagulation of retinal bleeding and retinal reattachment. This application of the laser can be delivered safely through the anterior part of the eye, since the laser beam passes through the cornea, lens, and clear vitreous, and is absorbed in the fundus oculi.

ND:YAG LASER

Neodymium:YAG lasers, which utilize as lasing medium a synthetic crystal of yttrium aluminum garnet doped with neodymium, generate coherent radiation at a wavelength of 1.06 μm. The lasing medium is excited or pumped by a flash lamp and can be operated pulsed, including Q-switched and mode-locked, or continously, with average power reaching 600 W. The efficiency of the system is, at best 3% to 5%, so it requires water cooling. On the other hand, low-power Nd:YAG lasers can be pumped by diodes with efficiencies of 5% to 8%, and these are air cooled; however, the lower power output in the range of up to 10 mW is too low for most medical applications. The Nd:YAG laser beam penetrates tissue and arteries to depths of about 5 mm and is very useful in deep-vessel coagulation.

The Nd:YAG laser can also deliver coherent radiation at a wavelength of 1.32µm, though at much lower power output. Since the absorption in water is stronger at this wavelength, as compared with that at 1.06 µm, this device is now being effectively employed in tissue welding in arteries.[1] A mode-locked Nd:YAG laser is used in ophthalmology for the removal of the posterior capsule of the lens, which is usually required subsequent to the removal of a cataract. The very short pulses, with duration on the order of a few nanoseconds, of the focused laser beam energy cause precise lesions within the eye by creating a microexplosion.

CO_2 LASER

The CO_2 laser generates coherent radiation in the infrared region of the spectrum at wavelengths of 9 to 11 µm, with the dominant one at 10.6 µm. It is the most efficient and powerful laser available, having up to 15% efficiency, with power outputs reaching 15 kW, making it the most widely used laser in industrial applications. The main advantage of the CO_2 laser is that its radiation is highly absorbed in water, and hence in tissue, to depths of less than a small fraction of a millimeter. This short penetration of the CO_2 laser energy causes it to function in a manner similar to a scalpel. The lasing medium is a gas mixture containing CO_2 and can be used in a flowing system, wherein the gas is continuously replenished, or in a sealed tube. For most surgical applications, the power output ranges between 10 and 100 W, and the laser must be water cooled. However, small, air-cooled CO_2 lasers, with power outputs at 1 W or less, have been employed in such applications as anastomosis.[2] An efficient method of CO_2 laser design has been to use the gas-containing enclosure in the form of a waveguide tube.

EXCIMER LASER

The excimer laser utilizes a medium of diatomic molecules consisting of a rare gas and halogen atoms. Since the diatomic molecule exists only in its excited state, it enhances the process of lasing. The excimer laser generates coherent radiation in the ultraviolet range of the spectrum. Typical wavelengths are 193 nm for argon fluoride, 248 nm for krypton fluoride, 308 nm for xenon chloride, and 351 nm for xenon fluoride. The laser's output is in the form of very short pulses on the order 1 to 80 nsec in duration, with energies of 1 J per pulse. The lasing medium is excited by a pulsed high-voltage discharge; its efficiency is 1% to 2% and it can be air or water cooled.

Unlike all other lasers used in medicine, which produce thermal effects in tissue, the excimer laser is alleged to produce photochemical reactions.[3] The ablation of tissue by the excimer laser is characterized by unusually clean and well-defined cuts. The use of excimer lasers at 248 nm radiation, which is strongly absorbed by DNA, may be contraindicated because of possible mutagenesis.

DYE LASER

Dye lasers are tunable in that they can produce coherent radiation over a range of wavelengths. The active medium is an organic dye in a liquid solvent and is optically driven, usually by another laser; e.g., an argon-ion–pumped dye laser can be tuned over the range of 400 to 1,000 nm, although several different dyes may be required to cover the entire wavelength tuning range. The dye laser is tuned by a special filter in the laser cavity.

Tunable dye lasers have been used in the treatment of port wine stains[4] and in the fragmentation of urinary and biliary stones.[5] Extensive use of the dye laser is currently being made in photodynamic therapy (PDT), which utilizes the unique properties of hematoporphyrin derivative (HPD). When administered systemically it is retained selectively by cancerous tissue. The substance is photosensitive, producing two effects. First, when excited by violet light at a wavelength of 405 nm, HPD fluoresces in the red region of the optical spectrum (620 to 690 nm). Second, when irradiated with light, usually at 630 nm, HPD undergoes a photochemical reaction, which results in the formation of a singlet oxygen and the subsequent destruction of the cell that retained the substance. The use of lasers in PDT is not mandatory; their use is indicated by the need to focus the light onto small-diameter optical fibers to deliver the illumination inside the body cavities and tissue.

It should be noted that the gold vapor laser, which produces radiation at 628 nm, has also been used in PDT.

HF AND E–YAG LASERS

The HF laser employs a low-pressure gas containing chemically produced HF and is excited by a high-voltage discharge. It radiates in the wavelength range of 2.6 to 3 μm. Its main advantage in medical applications is the fact that water absorption at the wavelength of 2.9 μm is considerably higher than at the 10.6 μm wavelength of the CO_2 laser, and that fiberoptic delivery systems, which

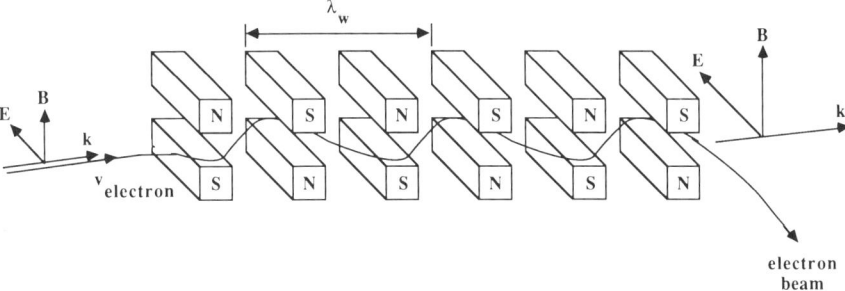

FIG 2–5.
Trajectory of an electron beam in a periodic structure of magnetic field in an undulator. N indicates north; S, south.

utilize fluoride glasses, are readily available.[6] However, the HF laser requires continuous pumping of the gas, and its exhaust is toxic. Instead, the erbium-YAG laser, which yields coherent radiation at 2.94 μm, is becoming the preferred choice.[7]

FEL

The medical applications of lasers utilize a variety of their features, as indicated above, i.e., diversity in wavelength, power levels, and pulse duration. A new type of laser, the FEL, provides all of the above features simultaneously over the widest range. Unlike all other lasers, which use a lasing medium, whether solid, liquid, or gas, the FEL derives coherent electromagnetic radiation from high-energy electrons in vacuum, which travel at velocities approaching the speed of light. These relativistic electrons are produced in accelerators and give up their energy in the form of electromagnetic radiation in special structures known as "wigglers" or "undulators."

Figure 2–5 shows the configuration of an undulator, which consists of a sequence of magnets producing a spatially periodic magnetic field. The electrons are deflected in the direction perpendicular to both the direction of the electron beam and the magnetic field. Owing to the spatial periodicity of the magnetic field, the transverse motion of the electrons follows a sinusoidal pattern. Since there is no increase in energy of an electron acted on by a magnetic field, the kinetic energy associated with its transverse motion obtains at the expense of the axial velocity. If an electromagnetic wave is superimposed alongside the electron beam such that its electric field component coincides with the transverse motion of the electrons, an exchange of energy between the two takes place. In particular, if the phase of the transverse motion of the electrons is slightly ahead of the electromagnetic field, the electrons give up energy to the electromagnetic wave, which thus experiences a gain. Figure 2–6 shows the arrangement of an undulator with mirrors outside the magnetic structure, which constitutes a laser resonant cavity.

LASER-BEAM DELIVERY

The use of lasers in diagnostic, surgical, and other therapeutic applications is greatly enhanced when employed in conjunction with flexible delivery of the laser beam, in particular if it is compatible with endoscopy. Laser-beam delivery depends on the wavelength of the laser energy, and at present there is no single delivery system that can be used over the entire range of medical lasers. The primary design considerations in such systems are efficiency, maximum power delivered, preservation of beam quality, and mechanical properties such as flexibility, degrees of freedom, range, size, and weight. Low efficiency (output power/input power) results in losses in the delivery system, which in turn requires higher power and thus more expensive lasers. Moreover, the power lost in the delivery system is generally dissipated as heat, resulting in a temperature rise that causes damage to the device, leading to a further deterioration of efficiency or catastrophic failure. Hence, efficiency, together with heat dissipation, can be considered to be the limiting factors in maximum power delivery. A well-designed laser oscillator emits a highly collimated beam of radiation, which can then be focused to a spot size of just a few wavelengths, yielding power densities not attainable with conventional light sources. A useful delivery system should, therefore, preserve this quality of the beam as much as possible; otherwise, the main advantages of using a laser are lost. The most desirable flexible system should be easy to handle mechanically and perform a large variety of tasks, while, of course, still satisfying the above properties. From a mechanical point of view, the ideal laser-beam guide would be an optical fiber of small cross section and long enough to reach any site, at any orientation, over a wide range of curvatures, through openings and inside complex structures.

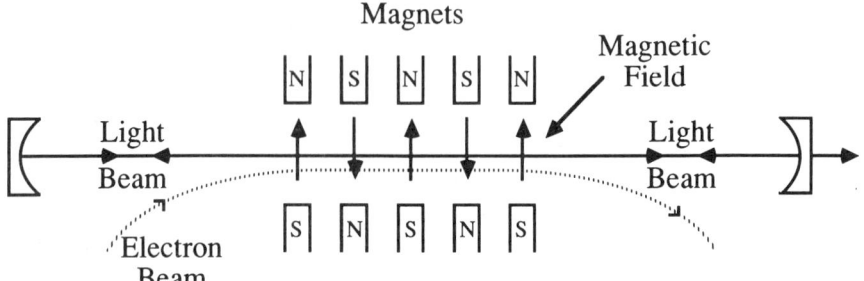

FIG 2–6.
Undulator resonant cavity in a free-electron laser. N indicates north; S, south.

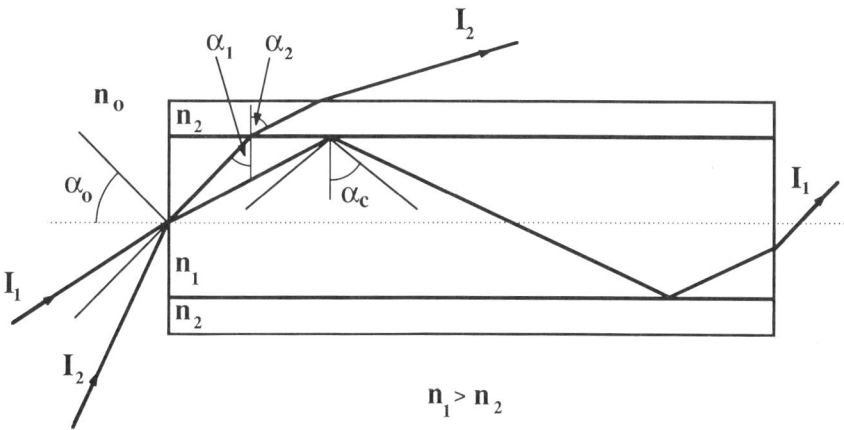

FIG 2–7.
Trajectories of meridional rays (l_1, l_2) in an optical fiber.

OPTICAL FIBERS

An optical fiber, which consists of a glass core and cladding, transmits light by total internal reflection. Figure 2–7 shows an axial cross section of a straight segment of an optical fiber and the trajectories of the meridional light rays. (Meridional rays, unlike skew rays, lie only in planes that include the axis of the fiber.) The trajectories of the rays are determined by the laws of reflection and refraction of light at the interface of two transparent media. The refractive index, n, which is defined as equal to unity for free space, is inversely proportional to the velocity of light in the medium and thus increases with the density of the material. The refraction of light at an interface between two media, 1 and 2, is governed by Descartes' law, which states that

$$n_1 \sin x_1 = n_2 \sin x_2,$$

where x is the angle between the light ray and the normal to the interface. In the transmission of light from a denser to a rarer medium of refractive indexes n_1 and n_2, respectively, i.e., $n_1 = n_2$, the ray is bent away from the normal. At an angle x_c, known as the critical angle and given by

$$\sin x_c = n/2/n_1,$$

the incident ray is totally reflected. In effect, the portion of light transmitted from a denser to a rarer medium diminishes rapidly for rays incident at angles approaching x_c and becomes zero at the incidence angle x_c. It follows that any ray, e.g., I_1 in Figure 2–7, incident at the interface of core and cladding at an angle larger than x_c will be totally reflected and will continue to do so repeatedly until it refracts and emerges at the exit face of the fiber at an angle equal to that at the entry. Hence, light entering the fiber within a given cone will emerge confined to the same angular pattern. However, if the fiber is used to conduct light into a fluid-filled cavity, as is often the case in medical applications, the refractive index of the surrounding medium is greater than in air ($n_o = 1.33$ for water), and the cone of exiting light may be considerably smaller than at the entrance, since the latter is usually in air. Light rays, whether partially or totally, are always reflected at an angle equal to the incidence angle.

Applying Descartes' law to the incoming light ray at the entry face of the fiber, corresponding to that which is internally reflected at the critical angle x_c, renders what is known as the numerical aperture (NA) of the optical fiber,

$$\mathrm{NA} = n_o \sin x_o = (n_{12} - n_{22})^{1/2},$$

which applies only to meridional rays. Since the transmission of light through optical fibers is mostly by skew rays, the actual NA is usually somewhat greater than that obtained in this equation. The effect of bending of the fiber on the NA is negligible since the length-diameter ratios are usually very large.

BEAM DELIVERY FOR VISIBLE AND NEAR-INFRARED LASERS

The representation of light propagation in optical fibers by rays fails to account for the phase differences in the optical path. The interference between the inclined rays (Figure 2–8) results in standing waves perpendicular to the fiber axis, which are known as waveguide modes. The modal theory of light propagation is based on the solution of Maxwell's equations within the appropriate boundary condi-

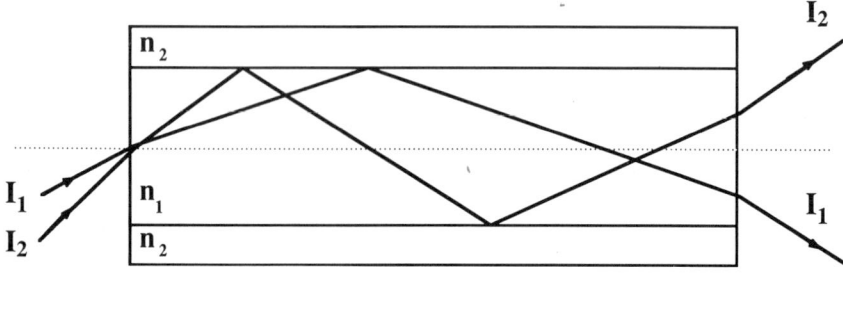

FIG 2–8.
Ray trajectories (I_1, I_2) in a step-index optical fiber; n_1 and n_2 are refractive indexes.

tions determined by the fiber structure and material parameters. As shown in Figure 2–4, light beams, in the lowest mode, emitted by lasers exhibit a gaussian distribution. To preserve the profile of such a beam, one must utilize an optical fiber that transmits a single mode only. In the case of a step-index fiber; single-mode operation occurs when the following inequality obtains[8]:

$$?d(n_{12} - n_{22})^{1/2} \; 2.4048.$$

Research in optical fibers for telecommunication has led to the development of glasses with extremely low loss (3% loss over a 1-km length of light transmission at wavelengths around 1.5 μm). Hence, such radiation when focused onto a very thin fiber (less than 1 mm in diameter) can be delivered at large distances with very little loss. When coated for protection, these fibers can be bent at radii of curvature of just a few centimeters. Single-mode fibers, which guide the radiation without affecting the beam quality, are currently being used in communications but to date have not been available for transmission of high power. The main reason is that their core is only about 10 μm in diameter and thus difficult to focus onto. So far, fibers with larger cores (0.2–1 mm diameter) have been employed; these do not preserve beam quality as well as single-mode fibers but have been found to be adequate in most medical applications. As far as power-handling capability is concerned, the typical glass optical fiber is quite adequate in applications where the laser-beam energy is delivered continuously or in relatively long pulses such that the peak power in optical fiber does not exceed power densities of several megawatts per square millimeter. However, when the laser energy is delivered in very short pulses, even a moderate energy per pulse may result in unacceptable levels of peak power. Such may be the case of Nd:YAG lasers, operating in a mode-locked or Q-switched configuration, which produce laser-beam energy in the form of pulses of nanosecond duration or less. In their current application in ophthalmology (capsulotomies), they do not require a flexible delivery system since the laser beam can be transmitted directly through the anterior portion of the eye. On the other hand, excimer lasers, which are becoming attractive in a number of applications,[3] generate energy in the ultraviolet range of the spectrum (200 to 400 nm) in very short pulses; they therefore require special optical fibers that can transmit light energy at such short wavelengths and, at the same time, carry the high power densities.

The energy of both the argon-ion and Nd:YAG lasers can be transmitted through optical fibers and thus directed through an endoscope. Indeed, both the argon and the Nd:YAG lasers have been used in the endoscopic treatment of bleeding ulcers.[9,10] Other endoscopic applications of the Nd:YAG laser, i.e., the transmission of its energy through optical fibers, includes vaporizing the interior lining of the uterus to destroy bleeding sites.[11] The use of lasers in miniature endoscopes has evolved primarily around their applications in cardiovascular diseases. However, the complexities associated with access, similar to those in angioscopy, and absorbency, remain to be resolved.[12] The combined features of a laser and a blade have been obtained in the design of a dielectric waveguide scalpel.[13] A beam from a 25-W argon laser is guided through an optical fiber to a fused silica scalpel blade. The blade forms a dielectric waveguide that carries the laser beam to a tapered cutting edge.

The limitation on power-handling capability of a glass optical fiber is due to several nonlinear effects such as Raman and Brillouin scattering,[14] avalanche breakdown,[15] and self-focusing.[16] Stimulated Raman scattering, which occurs when, due to molecular vibrations, a photon of one wavelength (say that of the laser) is absorbed and a photon of another wavelength (known as a Stoke's photon) is emitted, has been observed at power densities of 6 megawatts/sq mm. The time-varying electric field of the laser beam generates, by electrostriction, an acoustic wave, which in turn modulates the refractive index of the medium and gives rise to Brillouin scattering. Thus, Brillouin scattering is analogous to stimulated Raman scattering, wherein the acoustic waves play the same role as the molecular vibrations. Although the Brillouin gain is higher than the one measured for the stimulated Raman scattering, the latter is usually the dominant process in multimode fibers.[17]

Under the influence of an intense electromagnetic field, free electrons, which may exist in the optical fiber owing to ionized impurities, metallic inclusions, background radiation, or multiphoton ionization, are accelerated to an energy high enough to cause impact ionization within the medium. If the rate of electron production due to ionization exceeds the electron loss by diffusion out of the region, by trapping, or by recombination, then an avalanche breakdown may occur, resulting in material damage. If high enough power densities (above 100 megawatts/sq mm) are applied to the fiber core, avalanche breakdown is the main mechanism of permanent damage to the optical fiber. The fiber surface should be polished and chemically processed with great care to avoid reduction in the damage threshold level of the fiber surfaces. The latter is usually lower by two orders of magnitude than that of the bulk material owing to the presence of foreign materials embedded during improper polishing or owing to mechanical defects.

The threshold of induced Raman and Brillouin scattering and avalanche breakdown can be further substantially reduced by self-focusing of the laser beam. Self-focusing may occur when the refractive index of the nonlinear medium increases with beam intensity. The possible physical mechanisms involved are vibration, reorientation and redistribution of molecules, electrostrictive deformation of electronic clouds, heating, etc. Thus, a laser beam with a transverse gaussian profile causes an increase in the refractive index in the central portion of its path of propagation and becomes focused toward the center. Self-focusing is counteracted by the diffraction of the beam, and the balancing effects of the two determine the threshold of power that causes self-focusing; for glass it was found to be about 4 megawatts. Damage to optical fibers can also occur if a pulsed laser beam is not properly aligned with the entrance face of the fiber.[18]

BEAM DELIVERY FOR CO_2 (MID-INFRARED) LASERS

At present there are no optical fibers that can transmit the CO_2 laser beam, at 10.6 μm, as efficiently as it is being done in the visible and near-infrared spectrum. A long-standing solution to the flexible delivery problem at the wavelength of the CO_2 laser has been to use a number of highly reflecting mirrors (e.g., gold coated) that can be moved in concert to configure the optical path. Known as articulated arms, these devices consist of mirrors housed in boxes connected by tubes through which the beam passes without touching the walls. The tubes can rotate around their axis, thereby providing several degrees of freedom in the orientation and propagation path of the laser beam. The articulated arms have the advantage of preserving beam quality and of handling high powers. Their disadvantages reside in their relative bulkiness and possible lack of stability. Although very well balanced and with good maneuverability, articulated arms remain too large to be used with endoscopes. Also, misalignment of the mirrors can cause misalignment of the laser beam. This is particularly severe when the arms are used with a small handpiece, often resulting in the complete loss of the output beam. A modified version of the articulated arm consists of quartz tubings guiding the laser beam in its passage between the mirrors, which results in a smaller beam size[19]; however, the problem of mirror misalignment remains.

In optics, one can guide a laser beam tangentially along the inner surface of a concave sphere. To obtain a practical device, the circular shape of the guide can be made into a helix that can be extended without closing on itself. Owing to its coil-like shape, such a helical guide is mechanically flexible, allowing for the laser beam to be guided in various directions and distances within the limits of elastic deformation of the structure. The losses in the guide are measured by the number of turns or loops of the helical configuration. [20,21] Utilizing highly polished and dielectric-coated guides, it was possible to limit the losses to 5% per turn with only small increases due to stretching. The "whispering-gallery" waveguide can be used effectively in place of an articulated arm with the advantage of securing the path of the laser beam, which remains tied to the mechanical structure as though it were painted on it.

For the past 8 years, spurred by needs in military, industrial, and medical applications, the search for optical fibers in the mid-infrared region of the spectrum has been intensified. Crystalline, polycrystalline, and glassy substances have been investigated as possible materials for optical fibers capable of efficient transmission of CO_2 laser energy at 10.6 μm. The first successful attempt was the polycrystalline thallium bromoiodide, known as KRS-5, which is an optical fiber core about 1 mm in diameter obtained by extrusion.[22] Its transmission characteristics are excellent in the spectral range of 0.6 to 35 μm; at 10.6 μm, a 1.2-m long, 1-mm-diameter fiber can carry 40 W at a loss of 45% of its energy. However, the material is toxic and therefore requires special shielding, which is also necessary in view of lack of adequate cladding. It is commercially available at a very high cost.

Subsequent developments in polycrystalline fibers include silver bromides (AgBr) and silver chlorides, the latter serving as cladding to the former as core. They are pliable and, when fabricated by extrusion, can be produced at reasonable cost. Losses are on the order of several decibels per meter, which is higher than desirable, and the material is sensitive to light, particularly in the ultraviolet. Single-crystal AgBr have also been grown into fibers 0.3 to 0.75 mm in diameter, with a loss of about 7 dB/m. However, the rates of fabrication (2 cm/min) are too slow for efficient production. Other single crystals were also fabricated. Cesium bromide was grown into pliable fibers with a radius of curvature of less than 1 cm for fibers 2 mm in diameter. The fiber was able to carry continuously maximum power of 40 W at a 30% per meter loss. No cladding is as yet available, and the fiber was clad tentatively in Teflon. The growth rate, typical of crystal fabrication, was 5 to 10 mm/min. The fluoride glasses, such as Zirconium fluoride, have been produced with excellent transmission properties in the spectral range of up to 8 μm, which falls short of the CO_2 wavelength of 10.6 μm. On the other hand, a chloride glass, zinc chloride, has reasonable transmission at 10.6 μm; however, it is highly hygroscopic, making it difficult to consider for fiber applications. Recently, optical fibers made of chalcogenide glasses have again become the materials of choice for CO_2 laser-beam delivery. Numerous review articles have surveyed the developments in this field. [23,24]

The need for an effective beam-delivery system for mid-infrared laser energy suggests that other lasers be developed. For example, since appropriate optical fibers made of fluoride glasses are available, the use of lasers at wavelengths below 8 μm has been proposed. In particular, the use of lasers at 2.9 μm has been suggested,[7] wherein, as mentioned earlier, the absorption of water, and thus tissue, is even greater than at 10.6 μm, the wavelength of the CO_2 laser. On the other hand, attempts are made at developing miniature hollow metallic structures that can be made small and flexible enough to be used in endoscopy. To reduce losses associated with bending the waveguide,[25] the inner walls of the guide have been coated with appropriate materials, e.g., germanium, for 10.6 μm wavelength radiation.[26]

TISSUE EFFECTS

The effects of laser energy on tissue involve all aspects of interaction of light, albeit highly concentrated, with biologic materials.[27,28] The inhomogeneities of biologic tissue do not permit the development of a simple model of laser-tissue interactions, as the laser beam impinging on and penetrating the biologic materials undergoes complex scattering and absorption. Although most laser-tissue interactions are wavelength nonspecific, biologic tissues contain chromophores with significant absorptions in certain wavelength regions. The most significant absorber in tissue is water, its most prevalent constitutent. Other important absorbers are proteins, hemoglobin, and melanin.

The temperature of laser-irradiated tissue depends on the rate of energy delivered by the laser beam and the rate of heat dissipation, which in living tissue can be greatly enhanced by blood flow. When the laser energy is delivered in very short pulses, such as in Q-switched or mode-locked lasers, a sequence of very fast electromechanical events produces massive disruption of the tissue in the form of a plasma shock wave. Since the laser beam can be focused to an extremely small area, the mechanical events can be limited to a correspondingly small volume.

The understanding of the mechanism of laser-beam interactions with living tissue is of paramount importance to the future development of laser medicine and, indeed, is the subject of numerous current investigations. The complexities and difficulties encountered in formulating and solving this many-faceted problem will undoubtedly require considerable ingenuity and the recognition that only incomplete and approximate solutions may be possible.

REFERENCES
1. Schober R, Ulrich F, Sander T, et al: Laser-induced alteration of collagen substructure allows microsurgical tissue welding. *Science* 1986; 232:1421.
2. Quigley MR, Bailes JE, Kwaan HC, et al: Microvascular anastomosis using the milliwatt CO_2 laser. *Lasers Surg Med* 1985; 5:357.
3. Parrish JA, Deutsch TF: Laser photomedicine. *IEEE J Quant Electron* 1984; 20:1386.
4. Morelli JG, Tan OT, Garden J, et al: Tunable dye laser (577 nm) treatment of port wine stains. *Lasers Surg Med* 1986; 6:94.
5. Watson GM, Jacques SL, Dretler SP, et al: Tunable pulsed dye laser for fragmentation of urinary calculi. *Laser Surg Med* 1985; 5:160.
6. Wolbarsht ML: Laser surgery: CO_2 or HF. *IEEE J Quant Electron* 1984; 20:1417.
7. Wolbarsht ML, Esterowitz L, Tran D, et al: A mid-infrared (2.9 micrometer) surgical laser with an optical fiber delivery system. *Lasers Surg Med* 1986; 6:257.
8. Olsen RG, Rogers DA: Propagation in optical fibers, in Daly JC (ed): *Fiber Optics.* Boca Raton, Fla, CRC Press Inc, 1984, p 57.
9. Auth DC, Lam VTY, Mohr RW, et al: A high-power gastric photocoagulator for fiberoptic endoscopy. *IEEE Trans Biomed Eng* 1976; 23:129.
10. Silverstein FE, Protell RL, Gilbert DA, et al: Argon vs. neodymium-YAG laser photocoagulation of experimental canine gastric ulcers. *Gastroenterology* 1979; 77:491.
11. Fuller TA, Beckman H: Surgical applications of lasers. *Opt News* 1980; 6:20.
12. Isner JM, Clark RH: The current status of lasers in the treatment of cardiovascular disease. *IEEE J Quant Electron* 1984; 20:1406.

13. Doty JL, Auth DC: The laser photocoagulating dielectric waveguide scalpel. *IEEE Trans Biomed Eng* 1981; 28:1.
14. Stolen RH: Nonlinearity in fiber transmission. *Proc IEEE* 1980; 68:1232.
15. Bass M, Barrett HH: Avalanche breakdown and the probabilistic nature of laser induced damage. *IEEE J Quant Electron* 1972; 8:338.
16. Chiao RY, Garmire E, Townes CH: Self-trapping of optical beams. *Phys Rev Lett* 1964; 13:479.
17. Smith RG: Optical power handling capacity of low loss optical fibers as determined by stimulated Raman and Brillouin scattering. *Appl Opt* 1972: 11:2489.
18. Allison W, Gillies, GT, Magnuson DW, et al: Pulsed laser damage to optical fibers. *Appl Opt* 1985; 24:3140.
19. Bridges TJ, Strand AR: Waveguiding articulating arm for laser radiation. Read before the First International Congress on Applications of Lasers and Electro-Optics, Boston, Sept 20-23, 1982.
20. Marhic ME: Polarization and losses of whispering-gallery waves along twisted trajectories. *J Opt Soc Am* 1979; 69:1218.
21. Marhic ME, Epstein M, Kwan LI: Waveguide for surface wave transmission of laser radiation. US Patent 4,194,808, March 25, 1980.
22. Pinnow DA, Gentile AL, Standlee AG, et al: Polycrystalline fiber optical waveguide for infrared transmission. *Appl Phys Lett* 1978; 33:28.
23. Bendow B, Rast H, El-Bayoumi OH: Infrared fibers: An overview of prospective materials, fabrication methods and applications. *Opt Eng* 1985; 24:1072.
24. Harrington JA: A look at the future of infrared fibers. *Opt News* 1984; 10:23.
25. Marhic ME: Mode-coupling analysis of bending losses in infrared metallic waveguides. *Appl Opt* 1981; 20:3436.
26. Miyagi M, Hongo A, Aizawa Y, et al: Fabrication of germanium-coated nickel hollow waveguides for infrared transmission. *Appl Phys Lett* 1983; 45:430.
27. Welch AJ, Motamedi M: Interaction of laser light with biological tissue; in Martelluci S, Chester AN (ed): *Laser Photobiology and Photomedicine*. New York, Plenum Publishing Corp, 1985, p 29.
28. Grossweiner LI: Photophysics, in Smith KC (ed): *The Science of Photobiology*, ed 2. New York, Plenum Publishing Corp, in press.

3 Laser Safety

CAROLYN J. MACKETY, R.N.

Medical lasers have been used for therapeutic purposes for nearly 15 years on thousands of patients. In laser surgery, there are now more than 20,000 clinically documented cases. The number of known or documented injuries is less than 100, or 0.5%, in operations done with lasers.

This is a respectable safety record. However, the total number of surgical lasers in use today, worldwide, is unknown, although the potential market for lasers used in health care may be $76 million by 1987. In all specialties excluding cardiovascular, there are approximately 26,000 physician users for the various laser modalities.

As surgical and therapeutic lasers become more numerous and widely used by more physicians, the number of accidents is sure to increase, even if the rate remains the same. To avoid increased governmental intervention in medical affairs, and to avoid restricting the development of new medical lasers and new beneficial applications of this unique form of energy, it is imperative that every present and future user of lasers in medicine apply this promising medical device with the most careful regard for the safety of patients, physicians, and medical personnel.

Manufacturers must also bear their share of responsibility for the safety of medical lasers. They are now closely regulated by the federal government, as well as by state and municipal regulations for many classes of medical devices. As new and more sophisticated medical lasers become available, the manufacturers must carry the prime responsibility for educating the medical community in the safe and proper operation of their products.

Standards for safe laser use in health care facilities must be established to meet risk management and quality assurance patient care requirements. These requirements have been established by the guidelines, recommendations, and requirements of health departments and the laws that govern safe health care delivery. The following is a list (not exhaustive) of the groups and statutes that have been identified in the development of these guidelines: Joint Commission on Accreditation of Hospitals (JCAH); Bureau of Radiological Health; Occupational Safety and Health Administration; Industrial Hygienists; FDA; federal and state health agencies; medical device laws; American National Standards Institute.

The American National Standards Institute has established guidelines for industrial laser safety and has a committee developing laser safety guidelines for health care institutions. These guidelines, when approved and published, will be voluntary. Many of the medical and surgical specialties using lasers in their practice are beginning to address the special issues of safety. However, the hospital industry prefers to regulate itself with the established JCAH guidelines. There are no specific statements relating to a laser program, but the elements under risk management and quality assurance address safe practice as it relates to the use of hazardous medical devices. These elements include education and continuing education of the user, stated responsibility, policies or procedures, documentation of use, and preventive maintenance.

Each type of laser requires specific safety guidelines, as they are unique instruments that have been added to the physician's armamentarium. Lasers are considered hazardous medical devices and have been classified accordingly in class IV.

GENERAL CONSIDERATIONS

The invisible laser beams of the carbon dioxide (CO_2) and neodymium (Nd): YAG lasers are capable of inflicting third-degree burns. As a precaution against accidental exposure to the beam or its reflection, those using the laser should wear laser safety glasses as required. For the CO_2 laser, protection is also provided by any eyeglasses, plastic, glass, or prescription, that cover the whole eye. The safety glasses should have side protection for peripheral exposure. Do not use the surgical laser in the presence of inflammables or explosives; these include volatile substances such as alcohol, gasoline, solvents, ether, or any combustible anesthestic gases. A wet sponge should be inserted into the patient's rectum during procedures around the perineal area to prevent methane gas explosion.

The argon and krypton lasers used in ophthalmology, dermatology, and plastic surgery require eye protection of the correct optical density, as these lasers' wavelengths are in the visible range and can be refocused with the human lens and cause retinal damage. Also, the argon wavelength can potentiate photosensitive drugs, subsequently causing skin damage if these drugs are taken by the patient or staff.

Those who use medical lasers must always adhere to the following general rules:

1. Never operate any laser until you have read and understood the operator's manual furnished by the manufacturer.

2. Never fire any laser at any target until you know the complete path of the beam and are sure that no unintended targets lie in that path.

3. Never fire a therapeutic laser at any living target until you have been instructed by a competent teacher in both the correct operational procedures of the laser and the proper technique for application of the laser energy to the tissue to be treated.

4. Never use a laser for therapy until you have practiced its use on targets, cadaver parts, and laboratory animals.

5. Always take the safety precautions specified by the laser manufacturer when you use it for any purpose.

6. Never use the laser on human patients until you have taken a course of instruction in laser therapy.

7. Always request that a qualified instructor from the manufacturer give in-service training to the operating room personnel or laser support personnel in other clinical areas who may be using the laser, before use on humans. As the primary physician user, you also should attend the inservice presentation.

8. Always ask a qualified laser support instructor in laser operation to be present to advise you in your first therapeutic use of the laser on a human patient.

LASER SYSTEM SAFETY

To comply with the safety guidelines, each laser should include the following.

1. The laser should have a protective housing where the laser beam is totally sealed within the resonating chamber and output tube that leads to a shutter. No access is possible during the operation of the laser except at the output aperture. In a typical application, the output beam is totally enclosed all the way to the focusing lens. The resonating chamber forms a protective housing, and the laser tube assembly is covered to eliminate all collateral nonionizing radiation.

2. The key switch on the control panel is the master control. The key is removable only in the off position; the laser is not operable when the key is removed. The key prevents operation by unauthorized personnel and should only be available to the person in charge of the laser.

3. When the foot switch is activated, a light on the housing acts as a laser emission indicator. If illuminated when depressing the foot switch, it shows that power has been applied to the circuitry and laser output is available.

4. An electrically actuated shutter at the laser output provides a means for preventing human access to the laser output radiation without turning off the main power. The beam shutter is opened by depressing the foot switch. A manual safety shutter enables the blocking of the helium-neon (HeNe) whenever output is not desired.

5. Power monitoring is achieved through a built-in detector that measures laser beam power. The laser beam is deflected into the detector by the beam shutter when the power monitoring sequence is activated.

6. The device is labeled to certify compliance with standards that specify the power levels, laser classification, and location of the output aperture.

FEDERAL REGULATIONS

Laser equipment is very new in the medical field. As a device utilizing nonionizing radiation of electromagnetic energy, it is controlled by federal regulations. Some states are looking to establish regulations for nonionizing radiation devices. The following regulations governing nonionizing radiation are from the Occupational Safety and Health Administration (*Federal Register* 1979; 44 [Feb 9]:8589–8592).

A. Nonionizing Radiation

1. Only qualified and trained employees shall be assigned to install, adjust and operate the laser equipment.
2. Documentation of qualification of the laser equipment operator shall be available at all times and in the possession of the operator at all times.
3. Employees, when working in areas in which a potential exposure to direct or reflected laser light greater than 0.005 W (5 mW), shall be provided with antilaser eye protection devices.
4. Areas in which lasers are used shall be posted with standard warning placards.
5. Beam shutters or caps shall be utilized, or the laser turned off when laser transmission is not actually required. When the laser is left unattended for a substantial period of time, the laser shall be turned off.
6. Only mechanical or electronic means shall be used as a deflector for guiding the internal alignment of the laser.
7. The laser beam shall NOT be directed at employees.
8. The laser equipment shall bear a label to indicate maximum output.

B. Laser Protection

1. Employees whose occupation or assignment requires exposure to the laser beam shall be furnished with suitable laser safety goggles which will protect for the specific wavelength of the laser and be of the optical density adequate for the energy involved.

Lasers are controlled by the medical device law (21 CFR §1040), with four classes based on potential hazards that cause biologic damage. Lasers used in medicine and surgery are class IV medical devices. There are several subclassifications that require specific controls to maintain safe practice. Two values are set for the use of lasers in the health care environment. First is accessible emission limits or "maximum accessible emission level permitted within a particular class." Second is maximum permissible exposure (MPE) which is "level of laser radiation to which a person may be exposed without hazardous effects or adverse biological changes in the eye or skin." Criteria have been developed for MPE and are proportional for each wavelength exposure to laser systems with either pulsed or continuous wave.

Subsequently, medical surveillance should be performed as a baseline for all personnel working routinely with laser systems. This examination should be completed before employment and evaluated before termination or when a suspected laser injury has occurred. The components of the medical surveillance procedure include medical history with ocular emphasis; visual acuity, including a funduscopic examination; and dermatologic history, including medication usage, particularly those drugs that potentiate photosensitivity, which may be enhanced by certain laser wavelengths.

LASER USAGE AND THE LAW

Potential lawsuits concerning lasers fall into several categories: the allegedly negligent physician, failure to obtain informed consent, and corporate negligence of the facility for adequate supervision of credentialing. All medical personnel must be aware of the components of a malpractice suit: the "duty" or "standard of care" owed by health care providers to patients, breach of that duty or standard of care, and resulting injury or damages to the individual or proximate cause (causal connection between the breach and the injury). These components can be established by an expert witness in the course of the litigation. Another concern is the lack of consensus among experts in the laser field; however, the courts ultimately decide the standard of care.

What is the preceptor's liability? The preceptor may be liable for injuries caused by the student acting under his supervision. Guidelines for preceptorship must be established by the institution and approved by the medical executive committee.

If the equipment malfunctions, who is responsible? The health care provider may be liable for not making sure that the equipment functions properly. Risk management procedures should be established to assess unavoidable malfunctions and to determine strict liability through a negligence analysis. This analysis can be accomplished by using an "Accident and Malfunction" form, accompanying an incident report.

When lasers are used by physicians' assistants or nurses, state law should be checked for permissible activities. Each hospital should have written policies describing extent of supervision. The patient must be told who will be performing the procedure.

Informed consent requires adequate disclosure of the risks and alternative methods of treatment. Documentation of this communication is necessary, but the process of informed consent is more important than the consent form itself.

Minimizing liability by a well-defined safety protocol will reduce the risks, but the protocol must be carefully followed. Hospitals must establish a rigorous credentialing mechanism and uniformly enforce its requirements. A mechanism to review and consider regularly compliance with safety and treatment standards should be developed through the hospital's quality assurance program. Administrative controls for risk management include (1) development and approval of policies and procedures; (2) development and implementation of basic educational criteria for physicians and nurses; and (3) appointment of a laser safety officer, with the responsibility and authority for supervision of laser shutdown should a hazardous condition occur.

CREDENTIALING PHYSICIANS AND/OR NURSES

The *Accreditation Manual for Hospitals* (1985), under the chapter "Governing

Body," in several points discusses the requirements to assure that "all individuals who provide patient care services . . . are competent to provide such services." It also stipulates that "the quality of patient care services provided by these individuals be reviewed as part of the hospital's quality assurance program." A further requirement is "to implement and report activities and mechanisms for monitoring and evaluating the quality of patient care and to ensure "that all patients are receiving the same level of care."

The laser is representative of a class of medical instrumentation of complex and technologic advances where the user must be properly instructed in the use of this particular equipment. When the graduating resident or nurse has completed the study of lasers, including the biophysics, tissue pathophysiology, application, and safe use in practice, his or her credentialing certifies to his or her colleagues and the public a degree of recognized ability and expertise.

Credentialing controls access to difficult and complex instrumentation and techniques. The process of credentialing belongs within the institution and should be delegated to a multidisciplinary committee. The composition of this committee should be those who will use and maintain the instrument or technique in daily practice. The committee is usually formulated and directed by the facility's executive committee to develop written criteria and oversee approved regulations to ensure the safe use of the instrumentation or technique.

The recommended educational criteria could include (1) completion of an approved basic laser course that provides a stipulated number of hours for both didactic and "hands-on" clinical experience with laboratory animals, documented by a certificate awarded on the successful completion of the course; (2) participation in a preceptorship program in the physician/nursing specialty under the direction of an experienced laser physician/nurse either within or without the hospital's setting; documented by letter or form submitted on completion of the preceptorship criteria; (3) attendance at a formal in-service program conducted by the manufacturer on the operation and safety features of the laser and related equipment; (4) repetition of the above sequence should new laser systems be acquired; (5) if investigational lasers are purchased by the facility, the physician interested in using them should (a) submit a protocol for approval by the institutional review board or the human experimental committee; (b) follow the prescribed process developed by the principal investigator and/or the manufacturer; (c) provide special consent forms for the patient; (d) document the procedure; and (e) submit to the quality assurance or the peer review committee the appropriate data.

Nursing certification should be established in the same prescribed manner. However, there could be several additions for nursing credentialing criteria, including (1) development of standards for nursing practice during laser procedures; (2) development of a patient education process; (3) ongoing orientation developed for nursing personnel regarding laser safety; (4) nursing documentation of laser therapy; (5) development of a patient evaluation process; (6) establishment of discharge criteria.

Yearly random retrospective patient audits should be performed on those patients who have received laser therapy, by the quality assurance coordinator, to ensure that all criteria are being followed for laser practice established by the facility.

SAFETY GUIDELINES FOR THE CO_2 LASER

When using the CO_2 laser in the operating room, some special safety precautions should be followed.

1. The laser used not be used with alcohol preparations, ether, or combustible gases.

2. Safety glasses are required by all the operating room personnel, including the patient if she is under local anesthesia. The glasses may be plastic or glass and should have guards on both sides.* Half-glasses or contact lenses are not sufficient to protect the eyes. The laser beam may be reflected off shiny surfaces; subsequently, ebonized instruments should be used during the laser procedure.

3. Appropriate signs or notice should be posted on the operating room door, indicating the type of laser in use and the type of glasses that should be worn.

CONCERNS FOR SAFE OPERATION OF THE CO_2 LASER

The dangers in operating the CO_2 laser include the following. (1) The invisible beam can (a) ignite flammable materials, (b) inflict second- to third-degree burns, (c) be reflected, (d) cause severe eye damage; (2) the visible HeNe aiming beam can cause eye injury if directed into the eye; (3) the electric voltage used is potentially lethal.

ELECTRICAL HAZARD

The equipment is designed to limit accidental exposure to hazardous power. Use caution during service and maintenance. The following commonsense safety precautions should be followed: (1) disconnect power for all nonoperational servicing; (2) for operational check of the circuits, vacuum, and cooling system, ground all high-voltage circuits. No maintenance or servicing should be carried out with high voltage on.

---

*Protective eye wear may be purchased from Glendale Optical, 130 Crossways Park Dr, Woodbury, NY 11797; and from Eling Optical, Pleasant Street, South Natick, MA 01760.

MAINTENANCE

The overall maintenance of the laser is usually covered by a warranty or through a service contract. Laser equipment uses high voltage and emits laser radiation of high intensity. Any maintenance requiring removal of either the cabinet cover or the laser head cover or adjustment of the optical system should be done only by a qualified engineer.

Hospital preventive maintenance can easily be performed on the following components.

1. The *air filter*, located on the rear of the laser, should be removed and washed monthly with soap and water and allowed to dry before being replaced.

2. The *gas supply* should be checked after each use. Both laser and nitrogen cylinders should not be used if the pressure is under 100 pounds per square inch (psi). Outflow pressure of each cylinder should always be kept at 30 psi.

3. Before disconnecting the *gas cylinders*, be sure to turn the laser key switch off. Then close the cylinder valve and remove the regulator. When returning the laser to service, be sure to readjust the regulator for correct line pressure (30 psi).

4. The water level of the *cooling system* should be checked daily. The water level is indicated by the glass cylinder on the rear panel. Make certain the water level is between the minimum and maximum indicator marks on the glass. The water container is filled through the rear panel with distilled water as needed to keep the water level in this range.

All other problems must be referred to a qualified engineer.

SAFETY GUIDELINES FOR THE ND:YAG LASER

Operating room personnel should wear safety glasses with an optical density of at least 6 during endoscopic procedures. When using the Nd:YAG or visible lasers, all windows in the area should be covered.

The patient's eyes should be taped shut if he or she is under general anesthesia. Patients under local anesthesia should wear appropriate eye protection.

Appropriate class IV medical device laser warning signs must be posted on all entrances to the operating room or areas where the laser is in operation.

The designated laser safety officer should always be present during the Nd:YAG procedures.

Saline solution should be available during use of the Nd:YAG laser to reduce the possibility of heat buildup, particularly when the Nd:YAG hand piece is used.

LASER SAFETY RECOMMENDATIONS FOR AR AND KRYPTON

Argon and krypton lasers are in the visible spectrum, from 414 the pulsed Nd:YAG laser, in the near-infrared, is invisible at 1,060 primarily used in ophthalmology. For the YAG laser, another laser is coaxial aiming beam: the HeNe laser at 638 nm, visible light; or xenon light. Lasers used in ophthalmology cause injury to the target tissue with precisely controlled instrumentation. Argon, in the visible blue or green wavelength, is absorbed by hemoglobin or melanin and is used to photocoagulate leaking vessels in diabetic retinal disease. Krypton, with its wavelength at 618 to 632 nm (yellow, orange, red), is absorbed in the xanthophylls or the pigment epithelium and can be used in the macular area of the eye. The pulsed Nd:YAG laser used in ophthalmology uses a plasma shield causing photodisruption of the posterior capsular membrane. This wavelength, at 1,060 nm, is transmissible through clear or translucent material; it passes through the cornea and intraocular lens and finally opens up the membrane with no damage to the other ocular structures.

The safety policies and procedures that should be developed as applied to ophthalmology are as follows.

1. Appropriate signs should be placed on access doors indicating the type of laser in use, and access to the room should be restricted.

2. Eye protection of the correct optical density should be worn by staff, patients, and visitors, as follows: argon, orange/amber for greater than 488 to 514 nm; krypton, red/amber for greater than 514 to 618 nm; Nd:YAG, green for greater than 1,064 nm.

3. Viewing windows should be protected from wavelengths of 400 to 1,064 nm, which are transmissible through clear media. Shades, louvers, or green towels can be placed over the windows.

SMOKE EVACUATION CONSIDERATIONS

The CO_2 laser works by vaporizing tissue and produces a plume of smoke. As the operator vaporizes more tissue, smoke obscures the field and diffuses the laser beam. Though this smoke has not been shown to have biologic activity, its presence may keep the operator from accurately seeing the area to be lased.

Effective smoke removal is therefore necessary. Smoke can be removed by the internal vacuum system only if a filtering system is used. This filter should be about 40 μm and can be used in the line from the manifold and the suction canister. Suction canister filters are not adequate to evacuate the smoke plume. Vaginal speculums with smoke evacuator attachments are available; dental suction evacuators work well for ear-nose-throat cases, as does a rubber catheter along the endoscope.

Self-contained smoke evacuator systems are available and have internal filtering systems. Effective use of these systems requires proper filter maintenance, and they should be changed frequently. A room deodorizer can be used, or a small fan is appropriate in an enclosed area that does not have sufficient air exchange. The smoke evacuator should be turned on before the procedure and continue until all the smoke has been removed; this will minimize the odor in the laser room, which can be unpleasant.

ANESTHESIA SAFETY DURING LASER SURGERY IN THE UPPER AIRWAY

When surgery is contemplated in the upper airway, the known hazards and problems that existed before laser surgery are still present and must be considered. An obvious competition between the surgeon and anesthesiologist for control and space in the airway exists. Communication is necessary between the anesthesia care team and the surgeon. A plan for tracheostomy must be in hand before induction of anesthesia. Of course, when a compromised airway is known to exist, the patient should receive no preanesthetic medication that would depress respiration or increase the viscosity of the respiratory tract secretions. Such medication may be given in the operating room, where equipment and personnel are immediately available should resuscitation become necessary.

When laser surgery on upper-airway lesions is planned, the paramount problem is that of fire hazard. It is well known that if the CO_2 laser beam strikes an unprotected portion of rubber or plastic endotracheal tube, it will burn. The polyvinyl chloride (PVC) material produces an explosive fire, generally contained in the subglottic area or upper trachea. Burning will proceed distally with a torchlike flame as the anesthetic gases pass through the fire and support combustion. Hot foreign bodies, including portions of the endotracheal tube or aluminum foil tape, may be blasted into the distal airway and there produce local areas of high-intensity burn. Flame may also pass proximally and burn the lips and face. The larynx may be burned by heat transmitted from the endotracheal tube. In addition, the fumes produced by the burning PVC are toxic to the respiratory epithelium. There is probably some loss of surfactant within the lung, which may lead to atelectasis. The endothelial damage increases pulmonary capillary permeability, and potential for pulmonary edema at the alveolar level is coexistent with the loss of surfactant. Therefore, a PVC endotracheal tube should not be used.

Since the endotracheal tube must be in close proximity to the CO_2 laser beam, it is necessary to use measures that will diminish the probability of a calamitous fire in the patient's airway. Obviously, no ideal has been found as yet because there are many options available.

The endotracheal tube of choice is the red rubber tube, wrapped with aluminum tape. The selection of tape is critical. Lead tape is not acceptable. It is easily broken or melted and the vapors are toxic. There are reflective tapes that are nonmetallic and may have the appearance of aluminum tape. They are usually mylar tapes with a thin evaporated aluminum film. Mylar tapes reflect light but do not reflect the CO_2 laser energy and therefore will burn. A quarter-inch aluminum foil tape is wrapped in an overlapping manner from the proximal edge of the balloon to the edge of the bifurcation, making sure it is smooth and has no gaps. A water-base lubricating jelly may be used on the tube; however, I suggest lubricating with tap water. An oil-based ointment may be inadvertently substituted for a water-base jelly. Such an ointment can be ignited by a CO_2 laser pulse. A satisfactory alternative is the Norton tube, a flexible stainless steel endotracheal tube. This tube is relatively nonabrasive, totally noncombustible, and reusable.

Ignition of the endotracheal tube may occur in spite of the best efforts to prevent it. The severity of the subsequent injury to the patient will depend on the reaction of the operating room team. Proper, timely management is needed. Following ignition, immediately extubate and ventilate the patient with pure oxygen by mask. Continue anesthesia with a narcotic muscle relaxant technique to facilitate the necessary evaluation and management. Reintubate with a small endotracheal tube.

The surgeon should perform bronchoscopy and remove any remnants of the tube, tape, or other large foreign bodies. A flexible fiberoptic bronchoscope is then used to evaluate the distal airways and remove swollen particles of foreign matter. Examine the larynx and pharynx and excise any shreds of tissue that may be aspirated. A chest roentgenogram should be obtained soon.

It may be necessary to perform a tracheostomy. High-humidity ventilation is maintained because mucus plugs may form and secretions may be aspirated. Immediate consultation with a pulmonologist should be obtained. The needs of each patient will then vary with the extent of the injury.

LASER PERSONNEL REQUIREMENTS

Several specific positions may be required for the smooth operation of a laser program.

CLINICAL LASER NURSE

The clinical laser nurse participates in the perioperative role and in assessment, planning, implementation, and evaluation of the patient's care. The nurse assumes the responsibility for the direct supervision of other team members. She or he is responsible for the operation of the laser and its accessories, understands the maintenance requirements, and assists in developing and implementing the laser policies and procedures. The nurse is responsible for educating the patient and laser support personnel and orienting other employees to laser safety. The nurse is the assistant to the laser safety officer and has continued responsiblity to monitor safe laser practice.

In the selection of nursing personnel to work with the laser program, the following elements should be considered: maturity in judgment during patient care; education base to understand the significance of laser physics as applied to medicine and surgery; and reliability.

Nurses working with lasers should attend a fundamental laser educational course with didactic and clinical components. The educational components should include basic biolaser physics, tissue interaction, laser safety, applications of lasers and nursing interventions, and outcomes of laser procedures for patient information. The clinical component of the laser program should include operational characteristics, setup and shutdown techniques, care of laser accessories, and troubleshooting techniques.

LASER SAFETY TECHNICIAN

The laser safety technician works under the direct supervision of the clinical laser nurse and is responsible for setting up and shutting down laser equipment, observing safe laser practice, moving the laser, and following all laser policies and procedures. He or she assists during each laser procedure and may be assigned to run the laser during a procedure. The technician may be responsible for the care and cleaning of the laser and related accessories and equipment, and may document all laser procedures.

BIOLASER TECHNICIAN

The biolaser technician is responsible for maintaining the laser equipment and related accessories, including troubleshooting and minor maintenance for all laser systems. She contacts service representatives as needed for service or maintenance on the laser systems; assists in evaluating current laser equipment and may make recommendations as needed for accessories and equipment, and participates in in-service programs and orientation of personnel to laser safety and practice.

LASER SAFETY OFFICER

The laser safety officer should have the responsibility and authority for surveillance and implementation of the appropriate control measures to assure laser safety for the institution. This may be a full-time position depending on the number and placement of the lasers. The laser safety officer serves on the laser committee. The laser safety officer must have the knowledge and understanding of the technical mechanics of the systems, be able to assess laser hazards, understand the application of protective measures in the clinical arena, report all incidents, and plan for prevention of accidents. The laser safety officer should participate in the education of physicians and staff personnel during laser education programs.

Formal laser training programs have been established for physician and nursing education. When performing the laser laboratory exercises, all safety precautions for specific laser systems should be followed as outlined in the previous sections of this chapter.

As lasers proliferate in the practice of medicine and new laser technology is introduced, educational criteria, safety policies and procedures, and other necessary administrative responsibilites must be established. Laser diagnostic tools will be used in our daily practices; should there be potential safety hazards identified with the use of this technology, these will need to be addressed.

BIBLIOGRAPHY
1. *Laser Safety Guidelines.* American National Standards Institute, Z136.1.
2. *Laser Safety for Medical Facility: Preliminary Proposal.* American National Standards Institute, Z136.3.
3. Mackety CJ: Nd:YAG laser for posterior capsulotomy. *Today's OR Nurse* 1985.
4. Wallow IH, Myers FL, Kim YM, et al: Subretinal new vessels after krypton photocoagulation. *Arch Ophthalmol* 1985; 103(12):1844–1848.
5. Trokel SL: YAG laser ophthalmology. *Microsurgery* 1984.
6. *Guide for the Selection of Laser Eye Protection.* Toledo, Ohio, Laser Institute of America.
7. Norton ML, Simpson GT: Anesthesia management in laser surgery of the upper aerodigestive tract. *Ear Nose Throat J* 1982; 61:440–493.
8. Wrainwright AC, Moody RA, Carruth JAS: Anesthesia safety with carbon dioxide laser. *Anesthesia* 1981; 30:411–415.
9. Schramm VL, Mattox DE, Stool SE: Acute management of laser ignited intratracheal explosion. *Laryngoscope* 1981; 91:1417–1426.
10. Hermens JM, Bennett MJ, Hirshman CA: Anesthesia for laser surgery. *Anesth Analg* 1983; 62:218–229.
11. Mackety CJ: *Perioperative Laser Nursing: A Practical Guide.* Thorofare, NJ, Slack Inc, 1984.
12. Phister J: *A Guide to Laser in the OR: A Manual for OR Personnel.* Aurora, Colo, Education Design, 1983.

4 Anesthesiologic Considerations
TOD SLOAN, M.D., PH.D.

The introduction of technologic advances such as the laser into surgical practice provides improvements in the quality of patient care and surgical outcome. However, the optimal use of this technology relies on the assistance of the other patient care team members (operating room nurses and anesthesiologists). Clearly, these surgeries require the close coordination of activities of the neurosurgeon and anesthesiologist. This chapter will review for the anesthesiologist the various facets of operating room conduct and patient care that are affected by the use of the laser. These areas include (1) personnel safety; (2) patient safety; (3) management of the brain and spinal cord surface during laser application; and (4) implications for general neurosurgical anesthesia management.

PERSONNEL AND PATIENT SAFETY

As with all surgical tools, lasers present hazards for personnel in the operating room. As a concentrated form of energy, the beam of light can cause harm to all individuals in the operating room. For personnel, the greatest concern for harm from direct contact by the beam or reflected light is usually eye damage; minor skin burns are usually of less consequence. All individuals should wear protective glasses to prevent corneal or retinal damage. Fortunately, the most commonly used carbon dioxide (CO_2) laser is easily stopped by glass or plastic eye covering. Ruby, argon, and neodymium-YAG lasers require specialized eye covers designed specifically for their use. The patient's eyes should be closed and protected as usual. Since the patient will be unable to indicate inadvertent contact, tissue areas not necessary for the surgical field should be covered to prevent damage from reflected light or a stray beam.

Other hazards are a consequence of the laser energy. Potentially flammable items should not be used because fires and explosions can occur due to ignition from the laser. Thus, flammable anesthetics, paper, and flammable plastic drapes should not be used. Flammable solutions such as alcohol or colloidon should not be used before laser use. Finally, vaporized tissue fragments and smoke should be vented adequately to avoid contamination of the operating room environment.

Specific concerns also arise during operations near the airway, including transsphenoidal, skull base, or anterior cervical procedures. In addition to the usual concerns when the surgeon and anesthesiologist must share the patient's airway, there is the danger of inadvertent contact of the laser energy with the endotracheal tube. Perforation of the cuff of the endotracheal tube may allow aspiration around the endotracheal tube and may reduce ventilation. Contact with the tube itself can cause ignition of the tube and fire. The resulting fire, or toxic combustion products (particularly of plastic endotracheal tubes), can cause critical damage to the patient's airway. This problem is clearly more common for oral and tracheal surgery. A variety of protective measures have been employed in these latter situations, including wrapping tubes with metal foil, placing packing above the endotracheal tube, and utilizing metal tubes or rubber tubes that smolder rather than ignite.

MANAGEMENT OF THE BRAIN SURFACE

Second to personnel and patient safety, the neurosurgical application of the laser has its greatest implications for minimizing the motion of the surface of the brain or spinal cord. Movement of the surgical field must be minimized as much as possible for two important reasons. First, the surgical field is the target of the laser beam; movement of the field will cause damage to adjacent neural structures and may result in unnecessary destruction of critical neural pathways. Failure to minimize movement will thus degrade the precision of the instrument. Second, the laser may be utilized through endoscopes or with microscopes. With these optical devices, target movement may make microscope focusing difficult (if movement exceeds the depth of field of the optical system), and small movements will be amplified, making aiming of the laser beam difficult. Finally, small motion may defocus the laser beam. This may change a focused beam, intended for cutting, into a defocused beam that causes coagulation. Alternatively, a beam intentionally defocused for the purpose of coagulation may become focused and make a deeper incision than intended.

To minimize surgical field movement, the factors that can cause patient movement during surgery must be considered. These include (1) movement by the patient, (2) movement of the patient by operating room personnel, (3) movement of the brain and spinal cord secondary to ventilatory motion, and (4) motion of the brain and spinal cord secondary to arterial pulsations.

In the unanesthetized patient, coughing or voluntary muscular activity can cause gross movement. This is easily overcome by a sufficient depth of anesthesia, producing unconsciousness and insensibility to noxious stimuli. However, fluctuations in anesthetic depth and stimulation intensity may occur, resulting in patient movement. Therefore, a drug-induced state of neuromuscular paralysis is generally preferred. It is important to recognize that neuromuscular blocking drugs reduce muscular activity by blocking the neuromuscular junction, and that muscle activity will still result if the muscle is stimulated directly. This, however, is rarely a problem during neurosurgical operations, as the surgical field usually does not include muscle groups. Titration and redosing of these drugs is therefore important during the period when patient motion would be most detrimental using conventional neuromuscular blockade monitors. Furthermore, monitoring becomes important when resumption of neuromuscular function may be desirable, such as during craniofacial or posterior fossa operations to verify cranial nerve function.

A second source of movement is ventilation or other gravity-dependent factors that may cause the patient's head or spine to change position over time. To prevent this motion, the head, trunk, and limbs should be securely resting on padded surfaces. For intracranial, craniofacial, and cervical spinal procedures, the greatest fixation is achieved by placement of a pin-type head holder. For other posterior spinal procedures, resting the trunk on well-placed blanket rolls or a chest frame can securely hold the body. As pointed out in other reviews,[10] a variety of other factors are important in positioning for patient safety. Of particular importance in the prone position is maintaining freedom of abdominal movement; lack of free movement will result in greater trunk excursions during ventilation and a relative increase in blood flow through the epidural venous plexus of the spinal cord. This venous engorgement can cause increased congestion and bleeding in spinal operations.

Perhaps the easiest patient motion to control is that induced by personnel. This is primarily a problem when the operating microscope is in use, because minimal movement of the patient will be magnified. Prevention of this rests in placing surgical instruments and needed equipment away from the surgical drapes and patient. Furthermore, if the anesthesiologist needs to adjust the table or check the patient, it should be done at a time when motion will not be detrimental. Good communication between the anesthesiologist and surgeon is crucial.

The majority of the above patient movement can thus be prevented by the use of general anesthesia with neuromuscular blockade and common sense with positioning and patient contact. The remaining motion will be primarily the result of brain or spinal cord movement secondary to ventilatory motion or arterial pulsations. The largest fluctuations will probably be secondary to ventilation of the lungs. In operations of the spinal column, movement of the trunk is most critical. Here, careful positioning to allow free abdominal movement and the use of small tidal volumes will be helpful.

For operations on the brain, brain movement is less dependent on trunk movement and more related to the factors controlling intracranial volume. The contents of the cranial vault are the brain, cerebrospinal fluid, venous blood, and arterial blood. Only the last two volumes fluctuate rapidly enough to cause interference with the laser.

The most significant movement of the brain in the anesthetized and paralyzed patient is due to phasic changes in venous blood caused by ventilation of the chest. The change in intrathoracic pressure alters the drainage and volume of intracranial venous blood. Thus, with positive-pressure ventilation, rhythmic brain movement will be seen coincident with ventilation. Since the degree of movement will be directly related to the volume of venous blood and therefore to the degree of positive pressure used for ventilation, the largest movements will occur with large tidal volume ventilation.

The minimization of these ventilatory-related movements is related to the rate and volume of ventilation. Clearly, for extremely precise laser damage near critical structures, such as in the brain stem, the absence of ventilatory movements may be required. In this case, apneic oxygenation may be necessary. Here, the patient is ventilated with 100% oxygen and ventilation is ceased for the surgical lasing. With the patient's trachea intubated and 100% oxygen delivered, the Pa_{CO_2} will remain acceptable for some time.[6] However, the climb in Pa_{CO_2} will cause gradual brain swelling (due to cerebral arterial dilatation) and may cause cardiovascular stimulation with resultant increases in arterial pulsations in the brain. This technique can thus be used only for short durations of critical work.

Since ventilation must generally be continued during laser action, ventilation should be adjusted to minimize its effects. Rapid, shallow ventilation (respiratory rates of 15 to 20 breaths per minute) probably offers the greatest routine benefit. With slow, deep ventilation there will be periods of little movement with interspersed large variations. Although this technique may be valuable for other surgical techniques where the surgeon can time his activity to the breaths, the large excursions make the use of the microscope and continuous laser difficult for precision work.

The advantage of rapid shallow breaths is that movement, although present, is limited. This allows the surgical field to remain in focus (given adequate depth of field with the operating microscope) and limits the area of laser damage due solely to brain motion. The anesthesiologist must recognize that with shallow ventilation, each breath has a larger percentage of dead space ventilation, so that a larger total minute ventilation will be needed to maintain the same Pa_{CO_2} compared with slow, deep ventilation. Clearly, the use of end-tidal CO_2 monitoring or arterial blood gas determinations will aid in adjusting ventilation. In addition, the mean intrathoracic pressure will be greater under circumstances of rapid, shallow ventilation. Cardiac output may be slightly reduced by obstruction of venous return, and cerebral venous volume may be slightly increased. Monitoring vital signs and observing the brain will aid in optimal adjustment of these parameters.

Aside from apneic oxygenation and rapid, shallow ventilation, the use of high-frequency ventilation (ventilatory rates of 60 to 200 breaths per minute) may offer great advantage. Studies of brain surface movement in cats have demonstrated a reduction in surface movement to about one seventh that seen with conventional ventilation.[17] In addition, the phasic changes in intracranial pressure due to cardiac pulsations as well as ventilatory changes are less, particularly with reduced intracranial compliance.[2,12,17] The explanation for the blunting of the cardiac-induced movement is unclear,[8,9] but it is not due to a reduction of cerebral blood flow, which remains normal.[18]

These advantages, as well as advantages related to reduced intrathoracic pressure, reduced cardiac depression, and improved pulmonary drainage,[14,15] may make this an attractive method of ventilation when additional human studies are completed and ventilation equipment is more widely available. Ventilation at even higher rates (up to 40 breaths per second) may even offer additional advantages. At present, the preferred method of ventilation is rapid shallow breaths adjusted by monitoring the arterial or expired CO_2.

In summary, the reduction of brain or spinal cord motion secondary to ventilation of the lungs rests primarily on rapid shallow ventilation and monitoring of the expired or arterial CO_2. Ventilation by high-frequency techniques may offer some advantages but its practical utility in man awaits clinical trials.

A second source of brain or spinal cord movement is the rhythmic pulsation of the arterial vessel with each heartbeat. The fluctuation is due to the volume change in the arteries between systole and diastole of the heart. Aside from reduction of this effect by reduction in heart rate, the primary consideration is reduction of the arterial pulse pressure. Thus, it is important to review the essentials of hemodynamic physiology that determine the pulse pressure.

If we examine the factors producing the pulse, the magnitude of the rise with each heartbeat is a balance of the volume and force of the blood injected into the arterial vascular tree (the stroke volume) and the runoff of this volume into the vasculature (determined by the vascular distensibility and resistance). Minimizing pulse pressure is therefore achieved by decreasing vascular resistance and depressing cardiac stroke volume (by reducing cardiac contractility or preload).

When blood is ejected from the heart into the circulation, the pressure in the aorta that results is the product of the stroke volume and impedance to flow of the vascular tree. For a given stroke volume, the pulse pressure depends on the distensibility of the arterial vessels. As the vasculature is more compliant or distensible, less pressure results, yet blood flow will remain constant. Thus, for a given stroke volume, the reduction of pulse pressure requires an increase in arterial vessel compliance or a decrease in vascular resistance.

When considering vascular resistance, both the cerebral vessels and the systemic vessels are important. The systemic vascular resistance is primarily important because the total resistance determines the aortic root pulse pressure. It is this pulse pressure that has an impact on the cerebral vessels. Thus, attempts to reduce total vascular resistance by mild vasodilation will decrease the pulse pressure presented to the brain. This pulse pressure is then further modified in the brain by the interaction of the traveling pulse wave moving into the brain and the reflection of the previous pulse wave after it has interacted with the small blood vessels. Thus, the pulse in the small blood vessels of the brain may actually be greater than that of the aortic root (although mean arterial pressure remains the same). Since specific dilation of the blood vessels in the brain is contrary to the basic principles of neuroanesthesia, the only implication for management of the cerebral vasculature is that operations during cerebral vascular spasm may produce detrimental pulsations in addition to the reduced perfusion of neural structures.

Furthermore, since blood vessels are composed partly of elastic substances, as the mean arterial pressure is lowered and vessel diameter reduced, the vessels are relatively more compliant and pulse pressure is reduced. This latter effect may be less pronounced in older patients, where the replacement of elastic fibers by nonelastic collagen fibers makes vessels generally poorly compliant and pulse pressure greater.

Reduction of the volume of blood ejected from the heart will also reduce the pulse pressure. The factors determining the stroke volume are the afterload, preload, and cardiac contractility. Afterload was discussed above as the resistance to ejection of the blood. Cardiac contractility is the strength of contraction of the intrinsic myocardial fibers. In a normal heart, the contractility is governed by the balance of sympathetic and parasympathetic tones and the balance between catecholamines and other positive ionotropic substances with β-blocking substances. Contractility will be decreased by sympathetic inhibition, increased parasympathetic tone, and decreased catecholamine levels of β-receptor blockade. Anesthetic-induced cardiac depression will further decrease the contractility.

The relationship between contractility and actual stroke volume depends on the volume of the heart at the beginning of systole (left ventricular end-diastolic volume). This relationship is called the Frank-Starling relationship; there is generally an increase in stroke volume as filling of the heart increases. The factors that influence ventricular end-diastolic volume include ventricular compliance, atrial filling pressure, body position, venous tone, intrathoracic pressure, and total blood volume. Thus, factors that reduce venous return to the heart, such as raised intrathoracic pressure or reduced central venous volume, will decrease cardiac filling and ultimately stroke volume.

Since hypocapnia plays an important role in neuroanesthesia, it is important to consider the effect on pulse pressure. Since hypocapnia causes an increase in systemic vascular resistance and an enhancement of myocardial function, hyperventilation would appear to be detrimental in the reduction of pulse pressure. Studies demonstrate that the actual effect of hyperventilation is to reduce stroke volume and cardiac output, as well as to increase systemic vascular resistance. The next effect is that the deterimental effects are lessened.[4] In addition, if the pattern of ventilation used interferes with venous return to the heart (i.e., if it has increased mean intrathoracic pressure), the stroke volume and pulse pressure may be further beneficially affected.

In summary, the factors that favor reduced brain pulsations due to cardiac effects are (1) reduced systemic vascular resistance (such as mild vasodilation), (2) reduced mean arterial pressure, (3) reduced sympathetic tone, (4) low catecholamine levels, (5) increased parasympathetic tone or β-blockade, (6) cardiac depression, (7) decreased venous return, and (8) reduced circulating blood volume.

IMPLICATIONS FOR THE CONDUCT OF NEUROANESTHESIA

Several excellent discussions of the principles of neuroanesthesia are available.[5,11,13] Only the implications of the above considerations and other factors specifically applicable to anesthesia will be presented.

General anesthesia is generally preferable to regional or local anesthesia owing to the ability to prevent inadvertent motion at crucial periods of the operation. The ability to control ventilation using an endotracheal tube and the use of muscle relaxants clearly will produce a superior operative field. Good patient cooperation will clearly be necessary when operations are conducted using local techniques.

Anesthetic choices for general anesthesia should be based on the usual considerations for neurosurgery. A narcotic-based technique offers the advantages of mild bradycardia, reduced cerebral metabolism and blood flow, and increased airway tolerance at light anesthetic levels. Alternatively, light inhalational anesthesia with a volatile inhalational agent offers vasodilation and mild cardiac depression. With respect to the latter, isoflurane, an inflammable agent, may be the agent of choice owing to its reduced potential for increases of cerebral blood flow compared with halothane and enflurane.[3] As with the choice of major agent, the use of nitrous oxide depends on the basic considerations of neuroanesthesia. Of note is the potential for nitrous oxide to expand trapped volumes of gases in the brain; if pockets of air or vaporized tissue (steam) collect during laser endoscopic procedures, nitrous oxide should be avoided.

Monitoring of the neurosurgical patient undergoing laser neurosurgery should also be based on basic neurosurgical considerations. Of note is that, compared with electric or ultrasonic methods of tissue destruction, the laser produces less interference with monitoring devices. Thus, monitoring by electric methods is not affected by the laser. Perhaps the area of greatest advantage to the anesthesiologist is the lack of interference with sensitive electric monitoring. Of particular note is the lack of interruption to electrophysiologic monitoring (electroencephalogram and sensory evoked potentials) and Doppler ultrasound techniques used for detection of air embolism (one study suggests a reduced incidence of air embolism in the sitting position[7]). The patient with a pacemaker will similarly have less interference with the pacemaker. Finally, since electric current does not pass through the patient with the laser, the chance of electric burns is reduced.

Despite the precision of the laser, careful monitoring of the patient remains an important aspect of neuroanesthesia. Since a reflected laser beam or the heat absorbed adjacent to an area damaged by the laser may unintentionally affect a neurologic structure, the anesthesiologist and neurophysiologist must remain vigilant for signs of undesirable neural damage. For the anesthesiologist, this will be most important in the brain stem, where crucial cranial nerve and cardiovascular structures will be adjacent to desired neurologic targets.

For intracranial procedures, the usual techniques for reduction of intracranial pressure and brain bulk are equally valuable during laser surgery. Thus, hyperventilation, mild dehydration, elevation in positioning of the head, and reduction of cerebral blood flow favorably affect the factors discussed above to reduce brain motion. The reduction in cerebral blood flow will reduce the extent of edema known to occur in zones of tissue adjacent to the zone of laser destruction.[1,16] Reduction of the blood pressure in the surgical field will reduce vascular congestion and decrease bleeding, which can absorb laser energy, thereby reducing its effectiveness on desired tissue planes. This reduction in microvascular blood pressure will similarly allow the laser to produce hemostasis by thermal coagulation, particularly during laser destruction of vascular malformations.

At present the laser appears to have introduced no contraindications to anesthesia choices or techniques that are generally thought to be favorable in neurosurgery. The only major additional consideration is the attention to minimizing patient movement, primarily by using favorable ventilatory patterns.

CONCLUSION

The introduction of the surgical laser has been welcomed because it offers several advantages to intraoperative patient care. As outlined, there are several important considerations for patient and personnel safety from potentially damaging effects of a reflected or inadvertently directed beam. There are no major deviations from the usual tenets of routine neuroanesthesia management. However, simple adjustment of ventilation and cardiovascular parameters may reduce motion of the brain and spinal cord, improving the surgical field. The close cooperation of the anesthesiologist and neurosurgeon allows the surgeon to more fully utilize the microsurgical precision of this valuable tool.

REFERENCES
1. Ascher PW: Newest ultrasound findings after the use of a CO_2 laser on CNS tissue. *Acta Neurochir Suppl* 1979; 28:592.
2. Babinski MF, Albin M, Smith RB: Effect of high frequency ventilation in ICP. *Crit Care Med* 1981; 9:159.
3. Eger EI: Isoflurane: A review. *Anesthesiology* 1981; 55:559–576.
4. Foex P, Prys-Roberts C: Effect of CO_2 on myocardial contractility and aortic input impedance during anaesthesia. *Br J Anaesth* 1974; 47:669–678.
5. Frost EAM (ed): *Clinical Anesthesia in Neurosurgery.* Stoneham, Mass, Butterworths, 1984.
6. Frumin MJ, Epstein RM, Cohen G: Apneic oxygenation in man. *Anesthesiology* 1959; 20:789–798.

7. Jain KK: *Handbook of Laser Neurosurgery.* Springfield, Ill. Charles C Thomas Publisher, 1983.
8. Jonzon A, Oberg PA, Sedin G et al: High frequency positive pressure ventilation by endotracheal insufflation. *Acta Anaesthesiol Scand Suppl* 1971; 43:5–43.
9. Klain M, Smith RB: High frequency percutaneous transtracheal ventilation. *Crit Care Med* 1977; 5:280–287.
10. Martin JT: *Positioning in Anesthesia and Surgery.* Philadelphia, WB Saunders Co, 1978.
11. Newfeld P, Cottrell JE (ed): *Handbook of Neuroanesthesia: Clinical and Physiologic Essentials.* Boston, Little Brown & Co, 1983.
12. O'Donnell JM, Thompson DR, Layton TR: The effect of high frequency ventilation on intracranial pressure in patients with closed head injuries. *J Trauma* 1984; 24:73–75.
13. Shapiro HM: Anesthesia effects upon cerebral blood flow, cerebral metabolism, electroencephalogram, and evoked potentials and neurosurgical anesthesia and intracranial hypertension, in Miller RD (ed): *Anesthesia,* ed 2. New York, Churchill Livingstone Inc, 1986, pp 1249–1288, 1563–1620.
14. Sjostrand U: Experimental and clinical evaluation of high freuqency positive pressure ventilation (HFPPV). *Acta Anaesthesiol Scand Suppl* 1977; 64:5–178.
15. Sjostrand U, Ericksson IA: High rates and low volumes in mechanical ventilation: Not just a matter of ventilation frequency. *Anesth Analg* 1980; 59:567–576.
16. Smith A, Marque J: Anesthetics and cerebral edema. *Anesthesiology* 1976; 45:64–72.
17. Todd MM, Toutant SM, Shapiro HM: The effects of high-frequency positive ventilation on intracranial pressure and brain surface movement in cats. *Anesthesiology* 1981; 54:496–504.
18. Toutant SM, Todd MM, Drummand JC, et al: Cerebral blood flow during high frequency ventilation in cats. *Crit Care Med* 1983: 11:712–715.

5 Extra-axial Tumor Removal

LEONARD J. CERULLO, M.D.

Most neurosurgeons who have had the opportunity to use a laser removal of extra-axial tumors have been impressed by, if not convinced of, the usefulness of the instrument in this application. One can speculate that had meningiomas rather than gliomas been chosen for the initial clinical applications of the carbon dioxide (CO_2) laser in the early 1960s, the subsequent history of the laser in neurosurgery would have been drastically different. At present, it appears that the most widely accepted and uniformly appreciated use of the laser in neurosurgery is in the removal of extra-axial tumors of the central nervous system. These neoplasms offer the surgeon the opportunity to capitalize on the inherent gentleness and precision of the laser. Treatment of these diseases, histologically benign but frequently malignant by location, should be gratifying. Frequently, however, because of unexpectedly poor results, they leave surgeon and patient frustrated and angry. On the other hand, several series have now demonstrated that the use of laser for this group of patients has been rewarding. Statistically, patients do better immediately, are released from the hospital sooner, and enjoy a neurologically more normal life. When one considers that this group anticipates a full life expectancy, the neurologic status of the patient becomes all the more important from both a personal as well as a societal point of view.

The basic removal technique of extra-axial tumors of the brain and spinal cord is similar regardless of histologic variation or location of the tumor. There are, however, several nuances that relate to the type of tumor and its location as well as several surgical variations, both in terms of wavelength and technique. Both will be discussed after the initial principles have been elucidated.

The tumor is exposed through a modest craniotomy or laminectomy directly over the neoplasm, if this is possible. Ideally, the tumor surface, albeit minimal, can be appreciated from the surgical exposure without retraction of central nervous tissue. At this point, the arachnoidal plane between tumor and brain is identified and opened. It is critical to maintain this plane to avoid damage to surrounding neural and vascular structures and to completely follow the tumor through its often irregular course. The arachnoidal plane can be maintained open using moist cotton insinuated between the arachnoid on the outside and the tumor on the inside. During this phase of tumor preparation, careful attention should be paid to hemostasis and to avoiding mechanical trauma to the already severely compromised nervous tissue.

The CO_2 laser has been most widely used for the vaporization of extra-axial neoplasms and will be considered synonymous with "laser" during this discussion. Other wavelengths will be treated separately regarding their peculiar applications and indications. A site on the surface of exposed tumor is ascertained to be free from transversing neural and vascular structures. This site is chosen as the point of capsule entry. When the capsule of the tumor has been entered, the laser is used at low power to begin to vaporize tumorous tissue in an intracapsular fashion. Initially low powers are used, either intermittent or continuous, with a slightly defocused spot. This allows appreciation of the particular consistency and vascularity of the individual tumor. Each neoplasm is different in this regard, and further modifications of power density and radiant exposure are a function of the biophysical reaction of the particular tissue to this wavelength. The beam should be moved continuously to avoid drilling a hole into the tumor, perhaps precipitating bleeding in a location inaccessible without significant mechanical distortion of the tissue. Venous ooze can be controlled with suction while the laser is used to vaporize beyond the bleeding point. This will frequently result in excellent hemostasis without the use of other lasers or other tools for coagulation. Normally, the area closer to the capsule is more vascular, and bipolar cautery may be necessary to control the more active venous or arterial hemorrhage. Characteristically, extra-axial tumors are variegated in consistency. The particular area of tumor being dealt with will mandate the technical variations that are necessary for its vaporization. An attempt should be made to vaporize intracapsular tumor in a cylindrical or reverse conical fashion to keep the interior as open as possible while allowing the tumor itself to fall into the evacuated area. For large tumors, the laser may be used as a cutting loop with higher power and a more tightly focused spot to morcellate chunks of tumor in an atraumatic and hemostatic fashion. The geometry and size of the tumor will dictate the extent to which the intracapsular removal in this fashion is performed.

When an appreciable portion of the neoplasm has been so removed, attention is paid to the capsule. Using highly defocused energy at relatively low power, the capsule is irradiated. Depending on the collagen content of the particular tumor, the capsule will shrink to a greater or lesser degree. Shrinkage can be assisted by gentle massaging of the arachnoid over the surface of the tumor using moist cotton pressing against the capsule of the tumor rather than against the surrounding neural structure. The vessels that have been "swept away" by this procedure are normal vessels, whereas those that actually nourish the capsule can be coagulated either with the defocused laser or with the bipolar cautery. While the capsule is being irradiated and shrunken, the constriction of tumor will refill the previously evacuated intracapsular compartment. Occasionally, a nontumor vessel will be encased by neoplasm and can be appreciated at the surface. Meticulous dissection around the vessel, either with laser or with conventional technique, is necessary to protect that structure. On dissection, the vessel is flipped over or under the capsule, if possible, or protected with moist cotton if mobilization is difficult or dangerous. The location of vessels such as this can usually be appreciated with preoperative angiography. The plane, having been opened up between tumor and surrounding neural structure, is maintained using pledgets of cotton soaked in saline solution. This prevents neural tissue from falling into the working space, generally without relying on mechanical retractors. It also allows preservation and maintenance of the arachnoidal plane over the surface of the tumor. Finally, it prevents excessively deep penetration by allowing the surgeon to appreciate the limit to which he can safely vaporize tumor.

By alternating between intracapsular vaporization (or morcellation) and capsule shrinkage, the mass is eventually reduced in size. As the lesion becomes smaller and smaller, greater appreciation of the circumference, whether regular or lobulated, can be attained. As greater familiarity with the biophysical reaction of the particular tumor is achieved, higher-output energy can be utilized to expedite the process. When sufficient space has been purchased to allow mobilization of the tumor without mechanical distortion of surrounding neural structures, the vascular pedicle should be searched out and devitalized. This may be possible with laser of the same or different wavelength or with bipolar cautery. The devascularization of the pedicle of the tumor will frequently allow further shrinkage because of decrease in vascular engorgement and will make the laser vaporization more effective because of the loss of fluid in the tumor. On the other hand, the heat sink's beneficial effect of blood flowing through the tumor is minimized, and care must be utilized to avoid more deep and rapid penetration than had been previously noted.

The steps, then, of extra-axial tumor removal can be summarized as follows:

1. Exposure of tumor surface through a relatively limited craniotomy or laminectomy, centered over the most superficial and accessible portion of the neoplasm. Obviously, there are situations in which this is not possible;

2. Meticulous dissection of the arachnoidal plane between tumor and surrounding neural and vascular structures. Maintenance of this plane is essential to avoid damage to nontumorous vessels and structures and to allow complete removal of neoplasm;

3. Entrance into the tumor through the capsule at a safe area, free from transversing neural and vascular tissue;

4. Evacuation of the interior of the neoplasm (intracapsular removal) either by vaporization or morcellation of the tumor. Maintenance of hemostasis during this phase using either a YAG laser or bipolar cautery is essential;

5. Shrinkage of the capsule with defocused energy and continued preservation of the arachnoidal plane using moist cotton pledgets;

6. Continued alternation between points 4 and 5; and

7. Devitalization through vaporization or coagulation of the vascular pedicle and/or site of attachment; laser "sterilization" of this site.

Although the foregoing supplies a general rationale for extra-axial tumor removal, several specific variations may alter technique. Most notable among these is the specific location of the tumor.

CONVEXITY TUMORS

Convexity tumors with a wide base of dural attachment frequently have achieved significant size before they have been suspected and diagnosed. Accordingly, the benefit of a relatively accessible location is vitiated by the physical impediment of removal. Following circumferential incision of the dura as close to its attachment to the surface of the tumor as possible, arachnoid incision will isolate the neoplasm from surrounding brain. Defocused, relatively high-power CO_2 laser energy applied to the isolated dura will allow considerable shrinkage of the structure and will begin to "pull" the neoplasm from its nest. Small feeding vessels from the cortex can now be identified, coagulated, and divided. The surrounding cortex is then protected by moist cotton or gelatin sponges (Gelfoam), and the defocused laser can be used along the side of the tumor deep to the dural attachment to enhance shrinkage and delivery of the lesion. The process can be repeated as necessary until the entire lesion is free, or the tumor may be morcellated using focused laser energy as one would use a cutting loop. The more firm the tumor, the more impressive the shrinkage from defocused laser. The technique obviates the use of traction sutures and minimizes the risk of bleeding from ruptured or torn vessels deep in the tumor bed with potential for cortical damage. Morcellation, rather than vaporization, allows more speedy removal without the need for parenchymal retraction.

LATERAL SPHENOID TUMORS

Lateral sphenoid lesions are handled in a similar fashion, though it is frequently necessary to detect and to coagulate feeding vessels to the base of the lesion through the sphenoid wing. This is expedited by the use of the YAG laser at the base. Similarly, YAG or CO_2 laser can be used following removal of the mass to sterilize the bony attachment.

MEDIAL SPHENOID LESIONS

Medial sphenoid lesions present a greater challenge because of their involvement with both neural (first and second cranial nerves) and vascular (carotid, cavernous sinus) structures. Following appropriate craniotomy, the frontal lobe is elevated to expose the lateral-most aspect of the tumor. The superficial layers of the lesion are frequently quite friable and suckable, whereas the deeper tumor extending medially is more likely fibrous and punctuated by larger vessels. On incision of the arachnoid, the filmy layer is separated superiorly and moist cotton or Gelfoam is insinuated between the tumor surface and the overlying orbital frontal surface. This maintains the arachnoidal plane and prevents welding of arachnoid to tumor with loss of the plane. Superficial vaporization in conjunction with bipolar cautery or suction allows debulking of that portion of the lesion extending above the sphenoid wing to the orbital roof and planum sphenoidale. Following the tumor medially exposes the olfactory nerve superiorly and optic nerve inferomedially. This will frequently allow opening of the optic and the chiasmatic cisterns with the release of cerebrospinal fluid (CSF) and further decompression. The structures, having been identified, are protected with moist cotton.

Attention is now directed to the temporal base. The frontal retractor is released and the temporal tip is either displaced posteriorly by opening the sylvian fissure or elevated to expose the inferolateral extent of the tumor. During retraction, meticulous attention is paid to the vessels of the fissure, as the middle cerebral artery or its branches may be draped over the tumor and extend further laterally than would normally be anticipated. Strict attention to the arachnoidal plane will facilitate this maneuver. Vascular supply from the base and sphenoid wing can be dealt with using bipolar or focused YAG laser to isolate the tumor dome from its anterior and inferior blood supply.

The CO_2 laser is then used to vaporize lateral, then superior, neoplasm medially until the superior rise of the temporal base indicates approach to the cavernous sinus. At this time, attention is paid to the more posterior extent of the tumor. This is devascularized, then vaporized, in the same fashion until the tentorial notch is reached. The encysted ambient cistern is opened and CSF allowed to escape. This facilitates temporal lobe retraction in a superior direction and allows the tumor capsule to be pulled into the operative field after the arachnoid has been skimmed over the surface of the dome of the lesion.

Vaporization or morcellation of the posterior and superior extent of tumor will lead the surgeon anteriorly and medially. At this point, the cavernous sinus inferiorly and the carotid artery mediosuperiorly remain the only obstacles to complete tumor removal. Microdissection, following the vessels protected within the arachnoid plane, will terminate in the identification of the supraclinoid internal carotid artery. The tumor can be vaporized off the lateral aspect of the carotid, and microdissection will free neoplasm insinuated between the carotid and optic and third cranial nerves.

Similarly, manual dissection is required to extricate tumor that has extended through the tentorial notch, but at this point there should be adequate room for microdissection without the need for further retraction. A decision for complete removal or debulking will depend on the degree of carotid encasement, modified by the patient's age and clinical status. If complete removal is the objective, the tumor can be vaporized at low CO_2 power up to the lateral wall of the cavernous sinus. Adequate removal is evidenced by pulsation of the dural wall of the structure. Some would recommend YAG irradiation of the wall during continous cold saline irrigation to denature the tumor transmurally. This technique depends on the experience of the surgeon and should be weighed against the possibility of transmural damage to the carotid and cranial nerves. At completion, the base of the middle fossa and sphenoid wing are sterilized using CO_2 or YAG laser in the defocused mode.

PLANUM SPHENOIDALE TUMORS

Following appropriate craniotomy with exposure of the tumor, arachnoidal dissection isolates neoplasm from the inferior frontal lobe. Because of the tremendous variability and size of lesions in this area, as well as the optic nerve–chiasm complex vis-à-vis the superior or posterior limit of the tumor, general principles will be discussed. The initial debulking and devascularization of the tumor using CO_2 and YAG laser begins inferiorly and extends laterally before proceeding posteriorly. When a significant inroad along the base has been accomplished, vaporization or morcellation of the superior tumor for decompression can proceed in a safe fashion. Returning to the base, the surgeon may creep along the planum sphenoidale and lesser wing of the sphenoid until the ledge is reached. This requires tactile input and frequent monitoring. The ledge will herald the proximity of the optic nerve–chiasm complex and must be respected.

In the medial parasellar region, tumor is often seen extending under and lateral to the optic nerves with insinuation between the optic nerve and carotid artery. In this situation, inward collapse of the tumor is difficult because the lesion remains relatively stationary at its fixation on the planum sphenoidale and because of the tethering of the neurovascular structures. Tumor can be shrunken in volume by vaporization until the arachnoid plane between tumor and carotid artery and/or optic nerve has been identified. At this point, protection of these structures is possible and vaporization can proceed. Experience indicates that tumors in this region require more coaxing into the surgical field using microdissection techniques than in other areas of the skull base. Meticulous attention to laser technique is important to avoid damage by either direct or reflective laser energy. On the other hand, the ability to continually monitor visual evoked response recording while vaporizing tissue affords a greater measure of comfort to the surgeon and safety to the patient.

Following removal, sterilization of the tumor bed as previously described should proceed. In this situation, however, YAG laser is probably not to be chosen over CO_2 because of the risk of spread of thermal energy through the optic canal.

CLIVUS TUMORS

Tumors of the clivus will frequently extend to the opposite side, and a similar technique of tumor shrinkage with opening planes followed by protection is recommended. It should be remembered that laser cannot travel around corners unless deflected by mirrors, a practice that requires considerable skill and experience. Pulling on the tumor with pituitary forceps is just as dangerous, if not more so, and is not considered a suitable alternative for vaporization after protection. A transtentorial approach to these lesions is frequently desirable, and the CO_2 laser is found to be an excellent instrument for incising the dura when the inferior temporal cortex and superior cerebellar cortex have been protected.

FORAMEN MAGNUM TUMORS

The first step in removal of all extra-axial tumors following exposure is the identification and separation of the arachnoidal plane. This isolates the tumor from surrounding, often engulfing, neurovascular structures. If the lesion extends significantly into the spinal canal, laminectomy must be appropriately extended. Section of the upper dentate ligaments may allow the neural tissue to retract away while the tumor bulges into the operative exposure. Initial decompression is done using CO_2 laser to minimize thermal and mechanical trauma. The consistency and vascularity of the tumor dictate the most efficient radiant exposure.

Capsule shrinkage is an effective way to allow the tumor to dissect itself away from surrounding neural and vascular structures. This is performed with defocused CO_2 laser at lower power. Alternating between vaporization (internal decompression) of tumor and shrinkage of capsule allows the neoplasm to be dissected away from surrounding tissues and its site of origin determined. Although cranial nerve XI section has been recommended and is occasionally mandatory, it is usually possible to preserve this structure by removing the tumor from within rather than attempting to dissect it away en bloc. The generous clival tumor attachment is sterilized using defocused laser.

Tumors located at the anterior rim of the foramen magnum and extending superiorly or inferiorly pose the greatest challenge. Although the transoral route has been recommended, experience indicates that this is too confining in terms of surgical exposure. Consequently, the transmandibular approach is preferred. With the wide field offered by this exposure, CO_2 laser can be used either freehand with loop magnification or affixed to the operating microscope. The freehand mode allows great latitude in directing the beam into the more difficult-to-reach recesses of the exposure. This surgery, often extensive, is gratifying in terms of patient outcome because of its emphasis on exposure, minimal retraction, preservation of neural and vascular anatomy, and minimal trauma.

PETROUS TUMORS

The same essential technique applies to acoustic nerve tumors, meningiomas of the petrous bone, and other extra-axial tumors in the cerebellopontine angle. Following appropriate craniotomy with extension laterally to the lateral sinus and dural opening, the cerebellar hemisphere is gently retracted superiorly and medially. Frequently, drainage of CSF by opening the cisterna magna will aid in this maneuver. Usually, rather minimal exposure of the posterior aspect of the tumor is all that is necessary. Because of the deep extent of target and limited exposure, CO_2 laser affixed to the operating microscope is the ideal instrument. Conversely, visible wavelength lasers, such as the frequency-doubled YAG laser or the argon laser, can be used freehand and directed into the operative exposure.

The arachnoidal dissection proceeds as previously described. A point on the posterior aspect of the capsule is chosen and ascertained to be free from traversing neural and vascular structures. The capsule is entered at this point, and vaporization of tumor from within is begun. Initially, this is performed at low, slightly defocused power. As appreciation of the consistency and vascularity of the tumor is reached and radiant exposure is increased, though the defocused beam is found to be more effective than a sharply focused one.

When a significant portion of the neoplasm has been removed, attention is turned to the capsule. Again, using focused energy, the capsule is irradiated, and the tumor shrinks in circumferential dimension. The arachnoidal plane must constantly be verified and maintained using moist cotton or Gelfoam. Generally, exposure of the fifth cranial nerve superiorly or the lower cranial nerves inferiorly affords the first peek around the edge of the tumor. Debulking and capsule shrinkage proceed medially to identify the plane between cerebellum and brain stem on the one hand and tumor capsule on the other. The inferior medial extent of tumor dissection is often difficult because of the confluence of vascular structures, choroid plexus, and seventh-eighth nerve complex. Similarly, the supermedial extent is rendered difficult by the thinned fifth nerve and the often-encountered knuckling of tumor anterior to the brain stem.

When significant tumor has been debulked medially, the capsule can be folded in on itself. At this time, attention should be paid to the fact that the capsule of tumor may actually "accordion" or pleat and that cranial nerves anterior to the tumor can be captured in these pleats and inadvertently damaged. Accordingly, the capsule must be treated as a whole rather than piecemeal.

Rolling the tumor laterally allows identification, both visual and physiologic, of nerve VII. This structure can be protected while further tumor vaporization proceeds. The opening of the posterior wall of the internal auditory canal, if necessary, should be performed using conventional instruments. The CO_2 laser, however, is quite effective in vaporizing dura off the posterior petrous bone to expose the osseous structure, which is then removed using a high-speed drill with saline irrigation. Final remnants of tumor can be vaporized from nerve VII or manually dissected. If vaporization is chosen, very low powers and short exposure times are necessary to contain thermal energy. A small spot would be ideal with surrounding structures well protected with wet coton.

Extra-axial tumors vary in consistency and vascularity. As a general rule, the laser is the single most effective instrument for removing these neoplasms.

However, each case must be treated individually. Often, a very gelatinous tumor is just as well, if not preferably, debulked through suction or ultrasonic aspiration. The more sensitive the area, the more fibrous the attachment; the more firm the consistency, the better the CO_2 laser will function. Fatty tumors are particularly well vaporized because of the differential heat of melting of fat vis-à-vis neural tissue. In addition, the melted fat assumes a very low temperature because of energy absorption and will not cause further damage. It can be easily aspirated.

Though CO_2 laser has remained the mainstay of extra-axial tumor surgery because of its immediate absorption in water and minimal scatter, other wavelengths have been used adjunctively. The neodymium (Nd):YAG laser is most valuable in the devascularization of extra-axial tumors before their vaporization or morcellation with CO_2. Several aspects of the biophysical reactions of this wavelength of light on tissue deserve notice. As demonstrated by Burke et al., the maximal thermal conversion occurs beneath the surface. This has been used by Beck and Ascher in denaturing tissue beyond an intact structure, such as the dura of the sella or the superior sagittal and transverse sinuses. Because of this gradient in temperature elevation, however, an intratumor explosion, the "popcorn effect" described by Jain, can occur. Also described by Burke was the extension of damage, presumably thermal, to tissues beyond the margins of change demonstrated by histology. This zone of reversible altered metabolism, visible on histofluorescent techniques, widens the effective zone of YAG damage. This must be considered when using the laser anywhere near the interface between tumor and normal structures. It is contraindicated, then, to employ the YAG wavelength near the midbrain, the floor of the fourth ventricle, and the cranial nerves. The heat sink effect of tissue is compromised when Nd:YAG is used. The elevated temperature dissipates more slowly and temperature buildup is common. The applications of energy must therefore be of relatively short duration and modest power. This becomes more critical in dealing with tumors located in more sensitive areas.

It appears that the primary use of the Nd:YAG laser in the removal of extra-axial tumors is in the devascularization of the particularly bloody neoplasms, both in their center and at their vascular pedicle. This assumes, of course, that the vascular pedicle is not adherent to, or immediately adjacent to, sensitive and functioning neural structures.

The argon laser has been used for the devascularization and vaporization of relatively small extra-axial tumors. The low power of most available systems makes this wavelength, although theoretically very desirable, practically handicapped. The small spot size and coincidence of aiming beam with treating beam allow great precision and can be used to advantage in sensitive areas. It should be remembered, however, that the depth of penetration and degree of scatter are greater with argon than CO_2. The net result, as demonstrated by Edwards and

Boggan, is a lesion comparable in size with that of the larger spot CO_2. The availability of optical fibers to carry this wavelength and the ability of the argon laser to pass through clear media may make it ideal for extra-axial tumors in spinal fluid compartments such as meningiomas within the ventricular system. Again, however, the low power output of this relatively inefficient laser makes debulking through vaporization a relatively slow process. The frequency-doubled YAG laser, emitting near the argon green wavelength, may compensate for this shortcoming.

CONCLUSION

The surgical approach to extra-axial tumors should offer the following advantages: (1) immediate access to tumor with minimal retraction of already compromised neurologic tissue; (2) minimal thermal and mechanical trauma coincident with tumor removal; (3) preservation of normal arterial and venous anatomy to avoid vascular compromise at the site of the lesion or distal to it; (4) avoidance of cranial nerve sacrifice; and (5) complete tumor removal. Laser is the logical tool to achieve these ends.

BIBLIOGRAPHY
1. Ascher PW, Cerullo LJ: The laser in neurosurgery, in Dixon JW (ed): *Surgical Applications of Lasers.* Chicago, Year Book Medical Publishers, 1983, pp 163–174.
2. Bartal AD, et al: Carbon dioxide laser surgery of basal meningiomas. *Surg Neurol* 1982; 17:90–95.
3. Beck OJ: The use of the Nd:YAG and the CO_2 laser in neurosurgery. *Neurosurg Rev* 1980; 3:261–266.
4. Boggan JE, et al: Comparison of the brain tissue response on cerebral cortex. *Neurosurgery* 1982; 11:609–616.
5. Burke LP, Rovin RA, Cerullo LJ, et al: YAG laser in neurosurgery, in Joffe (ed): *Nd:YAG Lasers in Medicine and Surgery.* New York, Elsevier-North Holland Inc., 1983.
6. Cerullo LJ, Burke L: Use of laser in neurosurgery. *Surg Clin North Am* 1984; 64:995–1000.
7. Cerullo LJ, Mkrdichian EH: Acoustic nerve tumor surgery before and since laser: comparison of results. *JAMA,* submitted for publication.
8. Cozzens J, Cerullo LJ: A comparison of the effect of CO_2 laser and bipolar coagulator on the cat brain. *Neurosurgery* 1985; 16:449–453.
9. Fasano VA, et al: Observation on the simultaneous use of CO_2 and Nd-YAG lasers in neurosurgery. *Lasers Surg Med* 1982; 1:155–161.
10. Fox JL, et al: Lasers and their neurosurgical application. *Milit Med* 1966; 31:493–498.
11. Hara M, et al: Evaluation of brain tumor laser surgery. *Acta Neurochir* 1980; 53:141–149.
12. Hudgins WR: Use of the CO_2 laser in neurological surgery, in Snider WR (ed): *Laser Surgery Seminar: A Manual on the Carbon Dioxide Laser in Surgery.* Kansas City, Biomedical Lasers Inc., 1980.

13. Hudgins WR, et al: Microsurgical laser vaporization of inaccessible tumors of the central nervous sytem. *Dallas Med J* 1981; 76:245–250.
14. Jain KK: Complications of use of the neodymium:yttrium-aluminum-garnet laser in neurosurgery. *Neurosurgery* 1985; 16:759–761.
15. Kamikawa K, et al: Application of laser surgical unit in neurosurgery. *Surg Ther* 1976; 35:626.
16. Khromov BM, et al: Use of the laser in neurosurgery. *Vopr Neiokhir* 1974; 6:50.
17. Nishiura I, et al: Successful removal of a huge falcotentorial meningioma by use of the laser. *Surg Neuro* 1981; 16:380–385.
18. Perria C, et al: The CO_2 laser beam in the surgical treatment of cerebral tumors. *J Neurosurg Sci* 1979; 23:125–128.
19. Pimenta LHM, et al: The use of the CO_2 laser for the removal of awkwardly situated meningiomas. *Neurosurg Rev* 1981; 4:53–55.
20. Pimenta LHM, Pimenta AM: Evaluation of difficult placed meningiomas operated with CO_2 laser, in Kaplan I (ed): *Laser Surgery: Proceedings of the International Society for Laser Surgery*, Tel-Aviv, Israel, Ot-Paz Press, pp 147–148.
21. Rosomoff HL, Carroll F: Effect of laser on brain and neoplasm. *Surg Forum* 1965; 16:431.
22. Saunders ML, Young HF, Becker DP, et al: The use of the laser in neurological surgery. *Surg Neurol* 1980; 14:1–10.
23. Stellar S: Application of CO_2 laser to neurosurgical and other surgical problems, in *Proceedings of the Fourth European Congress of Neurosurgery*. Prague Avicenum Czech Medical Press, 1972.
24. Strait TA, Robertson JH, Clark WC: Use of the carbon dioxide laser in the operative management of intracranial meningiomas: A report of 20 cases. *Neurosurgery* 1982; 10:464–467.
25. Takizawa T, et al: Laser surgery of basal, orbital and ventricular meningiomas which are difficult to extirpate by conventional methods. *Neurol Med Chir* 1980; 20:729–737.

6 Pediatric Neurosurgery

MARION L. WALKER, M.D.

DAVID G. MCLONE, M.D., PH.D.

Lasers have easily and naturally found a place in the rapidly evolving subspecialty of pediatric neurosurgery. The immature and developing nervous system is especially vulnerable to the traumatic effects of surgery and to many of the traumatic side effects of treatment of the diseases affecting the nervous system of children. For this reason, minimizing trauma during the surgical procedure is especially important in pediatric patients. Although neurosurgery was somewhat late, compared with other surgical specialties, to implement the laser for clinical applications,[1,10,32,33] once neurosurgeons began to recognize the usefulness of lasers, pediatric neurosurgeons rapidly began using them in many varied applications.[3,6-8,20,37,39] This chapter will review the applications of lasers in the subspecialty of pediatric neurosurgery.

Many of the benefits of laser surgery that have been mentioned in other chapters of this book have special importance in pediatric neurosurgery. Certainly the minimization of blood loss in infants and children is important. Likewise, as noted above, the decreased trauma that accompanies laser vaporization of intracranial and intraspinal lesions is especially important in the child who still has a developing and maturing nervous system. The precision of laser surgery is an important part of this overall concept.

Though the laser can be either hand held or connected to the operating microscope, it remains essentially a microsurgical tool. Because of the qualities of precision and decreased trauma, the laser functions as a microsurgical instrument. It is most commonly employed with the operating microscope but can be used just as efficiently with the increased magnification of operating loops.

Although various laser modalities have been tried in pediatric neurosurgery, there has yet to be accumulated a significant volume of cases involving the neodymium (Nd) - YAG.[4] The FDA still has not released the Nd:YAG laser for general neurosurgical use and has been particularly reluctant to approve this laser for pediatric neurosurgery. There are, however, some institutions using the Nd:YAG in pediatric neurosurgical applications, and more information regarding its value will undoubtedly be available in the future.

Although the argon laser has been used in a number of neurosurgical applications,[3,5] it is not as common or as versatile as the carbon dioxide (CO_2) laser. References to laser use in this chapter will be to the CO_2 laser unless otherwise noted.

The laser is useful in treating several lesions affecting the developing and maturing central nervous system. Neoplasms of the brain and spinal cord have been especially vulnerable to laser removal, and it is in this area that the laser has had its most profound effect. This chapter will look at the effectiveness of laser surgery on various lesions in the brain and spinal cord, both developmental and acquired.

USE OF THE CO_2 LASER ON LESIONS OF THE BRAIN

CONGENITAL ANOMALIES

Congenital lesions (i.e., hydrocephalus, developmental cysts, encephaloceles) affecting the brain have not been found to respond well to laser surgical treatment. Currently, standard surgical approaches are more appropriate. Laser fenestration of cysts and intraventricular loculations through endoscopes is just developing, and the technique will undoubtedly be improved and become more widespread over the next few years. Congenital lesions affecting the spine have been treated successfully using laser surgical techniques. These will be commented on in more detail in the spinal surgery portion of this chapter.

VASCULAR LESIONS

As with congenital anomalies of the brain, vascular diseases have not yet been successfully treated in pediatric neurosurgery using lasers. This may be due to several factors. First, the CO_2 laser is not the appropriate instrument for treating most vascular lesions. Microwattage CO_2 lasers do have potential for treating aneurysms and vascular malformations but they have yet to be used in children. This, however, is a very promising area of laser use, and undoubtedly we will see future applications of this laser in pediatric neurosurgery. A second reason for the lack of laser treatment of vascular lesions in childhood is simply that vascular lesions are not nearly as common in children as they are in adults.

NEOPLASMS

The most intense use of laser treatment in pediatric neurosurgery has been in neoplasms of the central nervous system. The remainder of this section will discuss the laser treatment of tumors of the brain.

A discussion of laser treatment of brain tumors should include an understanding of the advantages and disadvantages of laser therapy. As previously noted in this chapter and elsewhere in this book, use of the laser will often result in decreased blood loss during the surgical procedure. The neovascularity of most pediatric neoplasms affecting the central nervous system is such that the laser seals the vessels as the tissue is vaporized, and blood loss is significantly decreased. This is observable even in lesions where one might not expect it to occur. Choroid plexus papillomas, for example, have generally been successfully vaporized using CO_2 laser therapy without significant bleeding, facilitating the debulking of the tumor centrally to allow easier and less traumatic access to the vascular pedicle.

The laser is most effectively used in treating tumors of the brain when it is attached to the operating microscope and used as a precision microsurgical tool. Standard surgical suckers or the Cavitron Ultrasonic Aspirator (CUSA) are often used to debulk tumors. Removal of the tumor and identification of the interface between tumor and brain is usually best accomplished with the laser. The laser allows easy identification of the tumor-brain interface in most cases.

The effects of laser on brain tumors can best be appreciated by dividing the tumors in terms of location and histologic type. We will discuss those tumors in the supratentorial compartment, noting the tumors found in the suprasellar region (including the optic pathway), tumors of the hemisphere, intraventricular tumors, and tumors in the pineal region. The discussion of posterior fossa tumors will include tumors of the cerebellum, the fourth ventricle, the cerebellopontine angle, and the brain stem.

Supratentorial Tumors

Tumors of the Suprasellar Region. — In childhood, tumors of the suprasellar region are most commonly gliomas affecting the hypothalamus and/or optic pathways and craniopharyngiomas. Although other tumor types may occur in this area, these two types are the most important for the purposes of this discussion. Gliomas affecting the optic pathway, especially those involving the chiasma and hypothalamus, are the most common tumors seen in this location in childhood.

Gliomas of the chiasma and hypothalamus, in our experience, are not usually treated successfully with laser surgical techniques. These tumors are invasive into the surrounding hypothalamus, and attempts at total removal are often devastating to the patient. Actual removal of all tumor tissue is rarely possible. For this reason, these tumors are generally debulked from their central portions using laser techniques, but rarely is the majority of the tumor removed. The biopsy is accomplished, and the patient is then either observed clincially or given radiation therapy. A surprising number of these low-grade neoplasms are very sensitive to radiation therapy, and the prognosis may be quite good despite the location of the tumor.

Craniopharyngiomas are generally treated quite successfully with laser techniques.[37] The central cyst can be evacuated, and the tumor attachments to the surrounding brain easily vaporized using microsurgical techniques with the CO_2 laser. It has been our experience that these patients can undergo gross total removal of the craniopharyngioma tissue with minimum surrounding trauma. We believe that microsurgical techniques, and in particular laser surgical techniques, have allowed more complete and less traumatic removal of these neoplasms than was previously possible. Patients we have treated in this manner have had better neurosurgical and neuropsychological outcomes than were previously described in the literature. Attempting total removal when feasible and avoiding radiation therapy provides the child the best potential for normal neurologic development.

TUMORS OF THE HEMISPHERE. — Tumors of the cerebral hemisphere can be treated by laser surgical techniques. It has been our experience, however, that these lesions are more efficiently resected using the CUSA. These tumors are usually adjacent to less delicate brain areas than other brain tumors in other locations and therefore can be successfully evacuated using the CUSA without injury to the surrounding brain. When there is an important adjacent brain area, the laser can help define the brain tumor interface much better than the CUSA in many circumstances.

VENTRICULAR TUMORS. — Tumors of the ventricle are often successfully treated with laser surgical techniques. These tumors are located deep within the brain, and the laser provides excellent access for tumor vaporization. Introduction of bulky instruments, such as the CUSA, into the ventricle is often difficult, whereas the laser allows easy and atraumatic removal of the tumor tissue. It has been our experience that this is one of the most appropriate applications of the laser in pediatric neurosurgery.

PINEAL TUMORS. — Tumors of the pineal region may or may not require an open surgical procedure. Our approach to these tumors has been to stereotaxically take a biopsy specimen of the tumor to obtain a histologic diagnosis. If the diagnosis necessitates an aggressive attempt at tumor removal, then the laser becomes the ideal tool. The laser allows vaporization of the tumor tissue in these deeply seated neoplasms. However, care must always be taken to avoid injury to important surrounding vascular structures.

POSTERIOR FOSSA TUMORS

TUMORS OF THE CEREBELLUM. — Tumors of the cerebellum may or may not be appropriate for laser treatment.[37] Cystic cerebellar astrocytomas with a small mural nodule are usually best treated by standard neurosurgical techniques. The tumor nodule can be removed easily and simply, and the laser does not afford any added benefit to the surgical procedure, unless the nodule is attached adjacent to important brain structures. Solid tumors of the cerebellum, however, are easily vaporized using the laser, and the atraumatic nature of this vaporization is especially important and valuable in tumors of the posterior fossa. We have found the laser to be especially valuable in those cerebellar astrocytomas that enter the cerebral peduncles. The point of interface between tumor and surrounding normal brain tissue can usually be identified so that a gross total removal is often possible even though the tumor extends into the cerebral peduncle.

TUMORS OF THE FOURTH VENTRICLE. — Tumors of the fourth ventricle include medulloblastomas, ependymomas, and choroid plexus papillomas. Although medulloblastomas may technically arise within the cerebellum, they are considered here as fourth ventricle tumors because of their location.

Medulloblastomas are usually easily suckable using the CUSA or the operating sucker. The margins of the tumor, however, are best treated by removing the tumor with the precision available from the CO_2 laser. Attachments of the tumor to the cerebral peduncles, the floor of the fourth ventricle, and the cerebral aqueduct are best removed using the CO_2 laser. Complete removal may allow the patient to enter a "good risk" protocol for treatment. In the infant, this may allow the patient to receive less radiation therapy to the whole brain.

Ependymomas have also been treated using the CO_2 laser. This tumor is usually very vascular and often attaches to the floor of the fourth ventricle. This attachment can be identified and the tumor tissue removed using the CO_2 laser. This requires experience in identifying the tumor attachment and then using the appropriate low wattage to avoid injury to structures beyond the tumor that are lying deep to the floor of the fourth ventricle, within the pons.

Ependymomas that are extending through the foramen of Luschka and into the cerebellopontine angle and anterior to the brain stem can also be successfully removed by laser. Attachments to vascular structures and cranial nerves can be vaporized. Again, however, it is important to have laser surgical experience and knowledge of appropriate power settings to attempt this type of surgical removal. Recent experience suggests that a more complete removal of these malignant neoplasms can be accomplished by using the CO_2 laser. This early experience also suggests that the outcome of these patients may be significantly improved when gross total removal can be achieved.[35]

Choroid plexus papillomas may occur in any portion of the ventricular system but are most commonly seen in the fourth ventricle in childhood. These tumors are vascular but, in our experience, are surprisingly well treated with the CO_2 laser. The laser vaporizes and seals all but the larger vessels. The tumor can be vaporized centrally, allowing easier access to the vascular pedicle before complete removal is achieved.

TUMORS OF THE CEREBELLOPONTINE ANGLE. — Tumors of the cerebellopontine angle in childhood include chroid plexus papillomas and ependymomas. The applicability of laser surgery to these lesions has been noted above.

Other tumors found in the cerebellopontine angle include exophytic neoplasms of the pons and the rare lesions affecting the fifth cranial nerve in patients with neurofibromatosis. Although the laser is valuable in the treatment of neuromas and schwannomas to this area, these are extremely rare lesions in children. Other chapters describe the technique of removing these lesions, and those techniques apply equally well in the pediatric neurosurgical patient.

Exophytic tumors of the pons extending into the cerebellopontine angle are almost without exception anaplastic astrocytomas or glioblastomas. Surgical removal does not change the rapidly downward clinical course of these patients.

BRAIN-STEM TUMORS. — One of the most important applications of laser surgical techniques to pediatric brain tumors is to those tumors found in the brain stem. Over the past few years, it has become apparent that the "brain-stem glioma" is not a uniform brain tumor but indeed is a collection of different tumors with different histologic appearances and biologic activities.[14,36,37]

It has been noted that gliomas of the pons can occur in several locations and have different clinical prognoses.[14] Those intrinsic tumors that infiltrate the pons are typically anaplastic astrocytomas or glioblastomas. These tumors have not been successfully treated with laser surgery; the patients have a rapidly deteriorating clinical course and rarely survive more than a year, even with radiation therapy and/or chemotherapy. Other forms of treatment must be found for these patients. Hyperfractionation radiation therapy is currently being evaluated and, at this early date, offers some promise for extended survival.[36]

Tumors of the pons that are exophytic into the fourth ventricle have a much different clinical prognosis. These tumors are often attached to the surface of the fourth ventricle and do not deeply invade the brain stem. They are low-grade astrocytomas and can be successfully removed down to their point of attachment into the pons. It now seems apparent that these exophytic tumors do not require follow-up radiation therapy, and many of these patients go on to have long-term survival without evidence of tumor recurrence.[13] Tumors of the pons that are exophytic into the cerebellopontine angle or anterior to the brain stem are generally malignant tumors and have a rapidly deteriorating clinical course. Lasers have not been successful in their treatment.

The area of the brain stem where tumors have been successfully treated has been something of a surprise. Tumors occurring in the medulla oblongata and at the cervicomedullary junction have been successfully treated with the CO_2 laser surgical techniques.[8,14,36,38] These tumors are almost always lowgrade microcystic astrocytomas. They are very similar to the neoplasms found in the spinal cord. Indeed, there are some who believe that these tumors may be extensions of upper cervical spinal cord tumors.

Surgical treatment of intrinsic astrocytomas of the medulla oblongata requires microsurgical and CO_2 laser surgical techniques. A posterior fossa craniotomy is done with the patient in the prone position to minimize the chance of air embolization. A midline opening provides adequate exposure. The posterior arch of C-1 is always removed, and occasionally a laminectomy of C-2 or lower is necessary. A standard suboccipital craniectomy is sufficient. Occasionally it is necessary to split the lower-most portion of the inferior vermis to obtain adequate exposure of the lower brain stem. The surgeon must be able to see up beyond the level of the obex, but an exposure of the entire fourth ventricle is usually not necessary. Tumors of the medulla that are surgically accessible will be below the obex and will present to the dorsal surface of the lower brain stem. Here the opening into the medulla is made to begin tumor removal.

The laser facilitates an atraumatic opening of the dorsum of the medulla. The tumor is immediately beneath the surface, and there is almost always a distinct border between tumor and normal brain. Using the CO_2 laser at low power settings, the tumor-brain interface can be easily identified.

Use of the CO_2 laser also allows for continuous electrophysiologic monitoring throughout the procedure. Spinal evoked responses and brain-stem auditory evoked responses are an important part of this type of surgical therapy. Although it is difficult to maintain spinal evoked responses when opening the dorsal surface of the lower brain stem, the brain-stem auditory evoked responses have proved to be extremely valuable. Even though the entry of cranial nerve VIII is about at the level of the surgical procedure, the surgery still has a direct effect on the brain-stem auditory evoked response. An increase in latency of wave I to V can be seen with retraction and also with heating of the surrounding normal brain tissue when the CO_2 laser is used. Removing the offending retractors or stopping the laser and irrigating the wound will return the evoked responses to their baseline. In almost all cases, the evoked response is improved at the end of the surgical procedure as compared with that noted before surgery.

The CO_2 laser appears to allow for greater tissue removal than that which can be safely accomplished using the CUSA. As noted above, the surgeon can usually visualize the tumor-brain interface quite distinctly, so it is not difficult for the surgeon to know the appropriate time for ending tumor removal. We have found the CUSA to be an effective instrument for debulking large brain-stem gliomas. The laser, however, is used to remove the tumor from the surrounding edges at the brain-tumor interface.

USE OF LASERS ON LESIONS OF THE SPINE

In spite of the continued controversy about what is or is not pediatric neurosurgery, a definite group of spinal cord lesions are identifiable as pediatric spinal disease. Beyond the obvious differences in size and blood volume, the child with a lesion of the spine presents a unique set of problems. Foremost among these is that surgery is indicated even though the child may be asymptomatic. In almost every case surgery is undertaken in the adult to relieve pain and/or a progressive neurologic deficit, whereas in children surgery is prophylactic to prevent infection or the onset of deterioration.[2,15,18,20,21] The presence of other lifelong handicaps, and surrogates — the parents — making decisions for the affected individual, further complicate this situation.

Certainly congenital lesions predominate in pediatric spinal disease, but neo-

plasms are not uncommon.[11] Fortunately, the majority of nec
able, and the outlook for independent function is good. T
where our approach has changed over the last 10 years. B
therapy were the preferred treatments until quite recently. Nu..
tumors can be removed without inflicting additional neurologic losses anu ...
the possiblity of restoring lost function.[6,7]

Use of the CO_2 laser substantially reduces the time required for surgery and the intraoperative blood loss, because the lesion is vaporized and small vessels are sealed simultaneously.[20] Only larger arteries require separate bipolar cauterization. This reduced blood loss is particularly important in infants with a small initial blood volume. Use of the laser also reduces the need to manipulate the tissues and the consequent operative trauma.

With magnification, the laser may be played over the exposed surface of the lesion, debulking it layer by layer. Loop magnification and the hand-held laser are preferred over the use of the operative microscope in large lesions of the spine, such as lipomeningoceles.[20]

This recent improvement in operative technique and in technology has led to reappraisal of the indications for surgery and the proper timing of surgical intervention. Large series now document that spinal cord lipomas can be untethered successfully and that the intramedullary portion of the lipoma can be debulked successfully with near-zero morbidity and mortality.[18-20] Furthermore, the series prove that such surgery leads to recovery of neurologic and urologic function in a significant number of patients with preexisting deficits.[20]

The rationale for intervening in asymptomatic patients is less direct but no less compelling. In brief, early intervention is effective prophylaxis against later, often irreparable damage. The time of onset or rapidity of progression of the deficit cannot be predicted. The common experience of pediatric neurosurgeons confirms that the decline in function may be either insidious or precipitous and that no schedule of routine follow-up can guard against interval loss of function. It is no longer tenable to advocate delayed or "cosmetic" surgery for this problem.

Finally, before discussing the various spinal lesions individually, one additional point should be made. The laser is a wonderful tool for preserving anatomic planes. The lack of bleeding and the laser's ability to vaporize loose connective tissue allows one to separate tissues and maintain their relationships to each other. This requires practice. Even more importantly, without understanding the anatomy on which you are operating, the laser will be of little value. As has been shown repeatedly, technology does not obviate the need for good surgical principles.

LIPOMENINGOCELE. — Spinal lipomas are masses of fat and connective tissue that have definite connection to the spinal cord and that may have attachment to the meninges. They are usually considered to comprise three subtypes: (1) intramedullary lipomas, (2) lipomeningoceles, and (3) lipomas of the filum terminale. These lipomas are believed to result from deranged neurulation, and an understanding of this embryopathy assists in dissecting this lesion.[20–22,24,29] The three subtypes of lipoma may produce symptoms in different ways. Intramedullary lipomas typically cause symptoms when the mass of fat compresses the spinal cord within the spinal canal. Lipomeningoceles and lipomas of the filum terminale appear to tether the spinal cord and lead to symptoms from cord stretching and ischemia.

Many, probably most, patients with spinal cord lipomas are neurologically and urologically normal when born.[15] An uncertain number, perhaps the majority, become symptomatic with time, and the percentage of symptomatic patients increases with age. Symptoms often appear during periods of rapid gain in height or in weight.

Treatment of spinal lipomas has been controversial. Many patients are asymptomatic initially, and although a few patients remain asymptomatic, the majority progress to irremediable neurologic and urologic dysfunction. All physicians have been concerned about the risks and the benefits of early surgical intervention. We recently reported the resection of a lipoma and untethering of the spinal cord in 50 consecutive cases personally diagnosed and operated on.[20] The 50 consecutive children operated on with the laser were taken from a series of approximately 140 lipomas operated on by one of us.

Our surgical technique begins with a midline skin incision with the knife, followed by laser dissection thereafter. The skin is then undermined laterally, taking care to leave intact a substantial layer of subcutaneous fat to provide the skin with vascular support.[19] The most cephalic intact neural arch is then identified by palpation. One to two levels inferior to this palpation indentifies the most cephalic widely bifid laminae and a distinct, tough, fibrous band that stretches across the midline to connect the club-shaped medial ends of the bifid laminae. This band appears to be a remnant of the tissue that should have formed the neural arch at that level. The band lies at the cephalic end of the fibrous defect in the spinal canal and tethers and kinks the dural tube, cord, and meningocele, which herniates dorsally through the fibro-osseous defect. One of the most important parts of the surgical procedure is section and release of the tethering band.

The next step in the surgical procedure is incision of the dura on the side of the widest subarachnoid space and away from the entry zones of the dorsal nerve roots. The widest subarachnoid space typically lies on the side opposite the lipoma and can be identified readily by preoperative sonography or magnetic resonance imaging (MRI). It is important to appreciate that the dura, the dorsal root entry zone of the placode, and the lipoma all come together at the same point. Although one is tempted to enter the subarachnoid space along the line at which the dura meets the lipoma, this is the worst possible place to do so, since the dorsal roots and dorsal root entry zone lie immediately subjacent to this line of junction. The best way to avoid this risk is to make the initial dural incision well lateral to the line of junction of lipoma and dura and at a more cephalic level where the anatomy is more nearly normal. Intraoperative sonography can be utilzed at this point to delineate the structures beneath the point of initial dural incision.[25,30,31]

It is important to perform a laminectomy as high as necessary to reach an area of dura that looks normal. The intact arachnoid can then be seen and, through the arachnoid, the dorsal nerve roots that pass toward their entry zone just beneath the dura-lipoma junction. This subdural space is an excellent plane to follow around the neck of the lipoma. Nerves do not traverse this space until they exit inferiorly. A small leaf of dura is left at the dura-lipoma junction.

The problem of visualizing the nerve roots and of getting lost following them through the fat is frequently alluded to in the literature. Nerve roots located beyond the lipomatous mass in the extradural location are in a normal fatty environment that does not represent a pathologic situation. Nerves in the subarachnoid space are not in the lipoma. The important thing to locate is the posterior margin of the dura.

Now it is necessary to remove the lipomatous mass that is adherent to the spinal cord. Once the dorsal root entry zone has been identified, the lipoma can be transected distal to that point. Occasionally the mass of the lipoma will anchor the cord within the canal and prevent simply transecting it. By playing the laser over the surface of the lipoma, the fat and areolar tissue can virtually be wiped away. It is possible to reduce the lipoma to proper proportion.

Care must be taken in removing the intramedullary portion of the lipoma. About 25% of lipomeningoceles have an extension into the central canal (Fig 6–1). This intramedullary component expands and thins the cord. A midline dorsal myelotomy may be required to move this segment (Fig 6–2). The exposed lipoma is easily vaporized, and a near-total removal can be achieved. There has been some controversy about the attempt to remove this intramedullary portion. It remains unclear to us why intramedullary masses anywhere else in the cord should be removed but not in the caudal end of the spinal cord. However, the interface between cord and lipoma is indistinct, making a true total removal dangerous.

At this point we begin closure by inverting the circumferential dural flap and subjacent pia-arachnoid over the distal cord and remaining lipoma (Fig 6–3). Because of the inversion, the smooth pia-arachnoid now lies superficial to the dura. The dura-pia-arachnoid flaps along each side are pulled together and overlapped to cover the distal end of the spinal cord with a smooth pial surface that, we hope, will reduce the incidence of retethering by scar. Previously, the

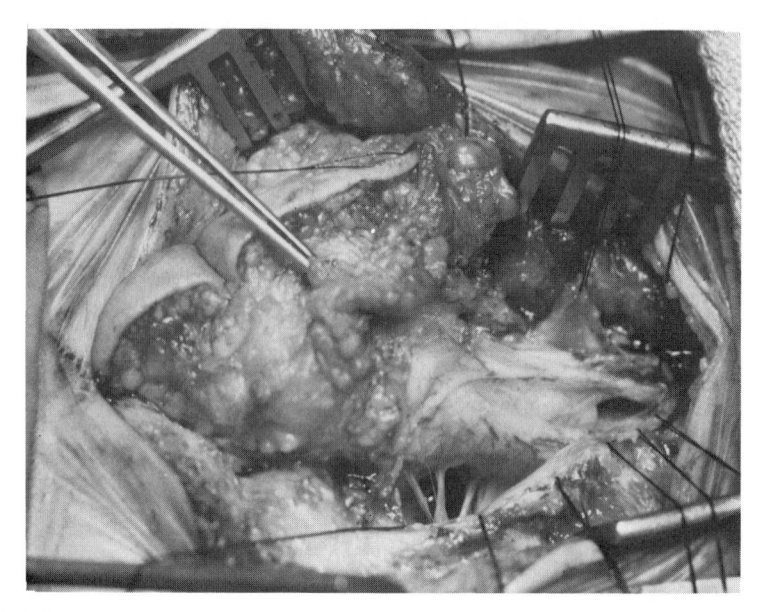

FIG 6-1.
A lipomeningocele with a significant intramedullary component. Fat is actually herniating through the dorsal raphé.

dural sac was reconstituted with fascia, but now a lyophilized dural graft is used to create a space that will distend with cerebrospinal fluid (CSF) and provide an environment in which subsequent tethering is unlikely.

Another technical point that deserves discussion is the case where the placode is tilted on its side. The dorsal and ventral roots on the deep side are unusually short. It is difficult to untether the cord in this situation, at least satisfactorily. The superficial side can be untethered well. The cord then moves well from side to side but not well in the rostral caudal direction. The short nerve roots deep in the canal fix the cord ventrally. We hope that those nerve roots will grow with time, thereby relieving the tethering effect.

We evaluated this technique in 50 consecutive children and had no mortality. No patient suffered increase in neurologic or urologic deficit. Postoperatively, 40% experienced substantially improved motor function. Urinary continence returned in 12%.[20]

DERMOID TUMORS AND DERMAL SINUSES. — Persistent attachment of the caudal end of the spinal cord to superficial ectoderm at the completion of neurulation allows a tract of squamous epithelium to be drawn into the spinal canal. With differential growth, the body trunk grows in length faster than the spinal cord, and the ectodermal tract is drawn rostrally as the cord ascends. This leads to two major problems: (1) the tract functions as a conduit to the outside world and a source of recurrent infection; and (2) portions of the epithelium become isolated and dermoid tumors develop. Because the attachment is filamentous, the cord is usually not tethered.

A couple of important anatomic points about the path of the dermal sinus tract should be made. Most descriptions state that the tract ascends from the skin dimple. We have now seen several cases in which the tract first descends one or two levels and then turns under the posterior spinous process and then may pass upward for several levels in the epidural space before it penetrates the dura. Once the tract penetrates the dura, one or more dermoid tumors may occur along its path. The tract will almost invariably end in the conus of the spinal cord. Thus, a multi-level laminotomy or small laminectomy will be necessary to reach the level of the conus.

The skin incision is made with a knife. An elliptical incision is made around the dermal sinus opening. The incision is extended rostrally to just below the level of the conus. From this point the laser is used to isolate and follow the tract to the point where it penetrates the fascia. The laser is used to incise the fascia and remove the paraspinous muscle from the posterior processes and lamina. Contrast myelography or MRI are useful to show the presence of dermoid tumors. If a tumor is present, a wider laminotomy or laminectomy will be needed

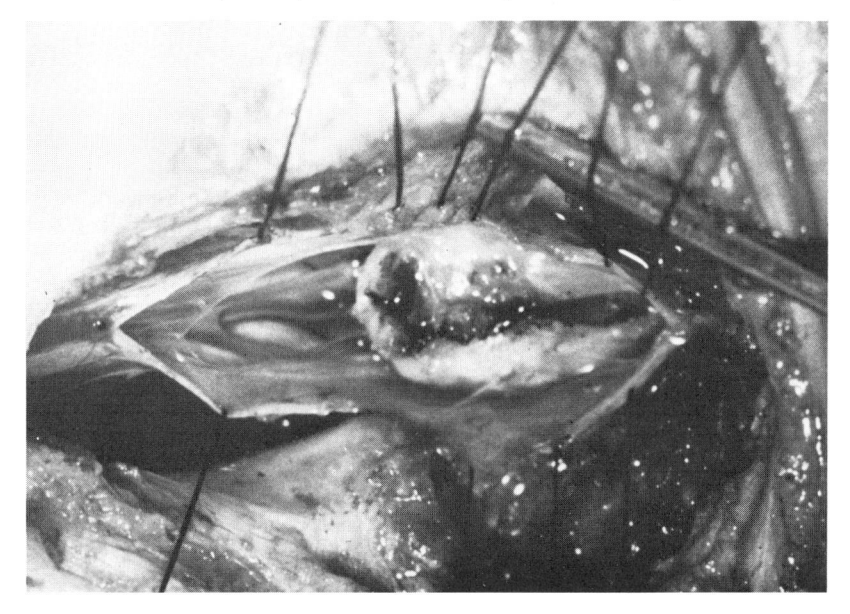

FIG 6–2.
The conus medullaris after a laser dorsal myelotomy and removal of the intramedullary lipoma. Note that the caudal spinal cord is now untethered.

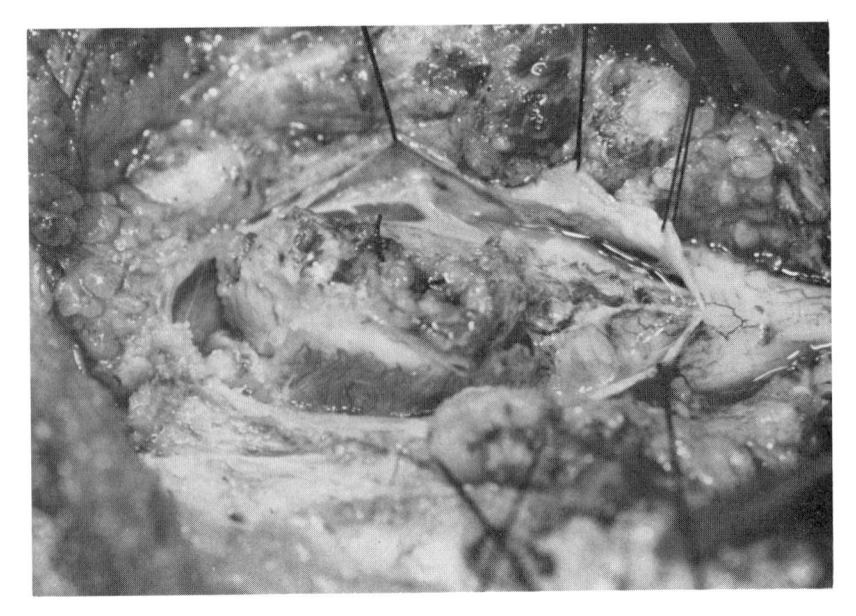

FIG 6–3.
Pial sutures are used to reduce the amount of rare tissue that might adhere to the dural closure. A dural graft was then used to establish a generous subarachnoid space.

at that level. If the tumor is adherent to the nerves of the cauda equina, the laser at low wattage is excellent for removing fragments of tumor. The tract must be followed to the conus, and the laser is used to resect the attachment to neural tissue.

TETHERED CORD. — Fixation of the caudal spinal cord often leads to gradual deterioration in spinal cord function.[12,31] This distal tethering of the spinal cord results in tension within the cord as it is "bow-stringed" between two points of fixation, the brain and conus. Stretch of the spinal cord causes increased medullary pressure and decreased caliber of vessels within the cord. The spinal cord is subjected to repeated episodes of ischemia and deteriorates over time.[40] The causes of tethering are numerous, but the mechanisms of progressive cord dysfunction are thought to be the same.

Tethered cord can result from a defect in regression of the distal neural tube in early embryonic life. A thickened filum terminale ties the distal cord in the sacrum and does not allow the normal ascent of the conus to upper lumbar levels during fetal life. Lipomeningocele, myelomeningocele, myelocystocele, dermal sinuses, and diastematomyelia are some of the other causes of tethering.[17,18,20,23,26] It is important to remember that scar formation following the repair of any of these lesions can cause retethering of the cord and necessitate reoperation to release the cord.

Changes in bladder and bowel function, gait, and strength are common manifestations of a tethered cord. Atrophy and/or a progressive foot deformity are often seen in younger children. Pain is one of the hallmarks of tethering and may be the only complaint. Pain is almost always relieved by surgery, whereas motor function has a 50% chance of improving and bladder and bowel function a 10% to 15% chance of improving. When atrophy is present, it usually persists. The technique is essentialy the same as those mentioned in the previous two sections.

MYELOMENINGOCELE. — The ramifications and nuances of this complex disorder are beyond the scope of this chapter.[17,19] What needs to be stressed here is that the initial technique for repair of the myelomeningocele is important to preserve function and prevent tethering later. The laser can be useful in this repair.

The technique for repair of the myelomeningocele has been detailed in another publication. The important steps in the repair where the laser is useful are the initial dissection of the placode, mobilization of the dura mater, and isolation of fascial flaps to cover the closure.

Dissection of the edge of the placode at the interface with the thin epithelium that extends out from the normal skin is the first important step (Fig 6–4). Failure to remove all of the epithelium from the placode will allow epithelial cells to be incorporated into the closure and lead to the formation of an inclusion dermoid tumor. Magnification and the laser at low wattage enable the surgeon to vaporize the epithelium and establish a clean edge along the placode.

The next step is to free the dura from the undersurface of the surrounding skin. By using the laser, the precise junction can be incised and bleeding in the epidural fat obviated (Fig 6–5). All of the available dura can be mobilized with near-zero blood loss. This allows a watertight closure and preserves the critical blood volume of the newborn.

Finally, a fascial flap from either side is turned over the closure to reinforce it (Fig 6–6). The dissection of these flaps with any other instrument is difficult and often leads to significant blood loss. The laser cuts a bloodless plane through muscle under the fascia and easily frees the fascia from its insertion along the ileac crest. The two well-vascularized flaps can then be folded over the closure.

CHIARI II DEFORMITY. — This complex malformation is almost always associated with myelomeningocele.[27] Although more is involved, the portion that is located within the cervical spinal canal will be discussed here. The foramen magnum is usually large, and a vermian segment of the cerebellum extends for a variable distance into the cervical canal. The cerebellum literally sits on the posterior arch of the first vertebra and has a portion of the vermis that can extend down as low as C-7. The cervicomedullary junction accompanies this vermian peg into the cervical canal and, therefore, so does the fourth ventricle.

Entrapment and compression of these structures are thought to lead to a variety of problems that afflict individuals with the II Chiari malformation. Apnea, vocal cord paralysis, absent gag reflex, gastric reflux with aspiration, and impaired upper-extremity motor function are some of the problems.[9,34] Cervical decompression (posterior fossa decompression) has been employed in the hope that relieving the compression would allow recovery of function. This has been followed with variable success. Certainly in older children it has been lifesaving. The controversy surrounds its benefit in the neonate.[19]

The lateral or prone position is usually used. A midline skin incision extends from the external occipital protuberance to the lower cervical segments. The

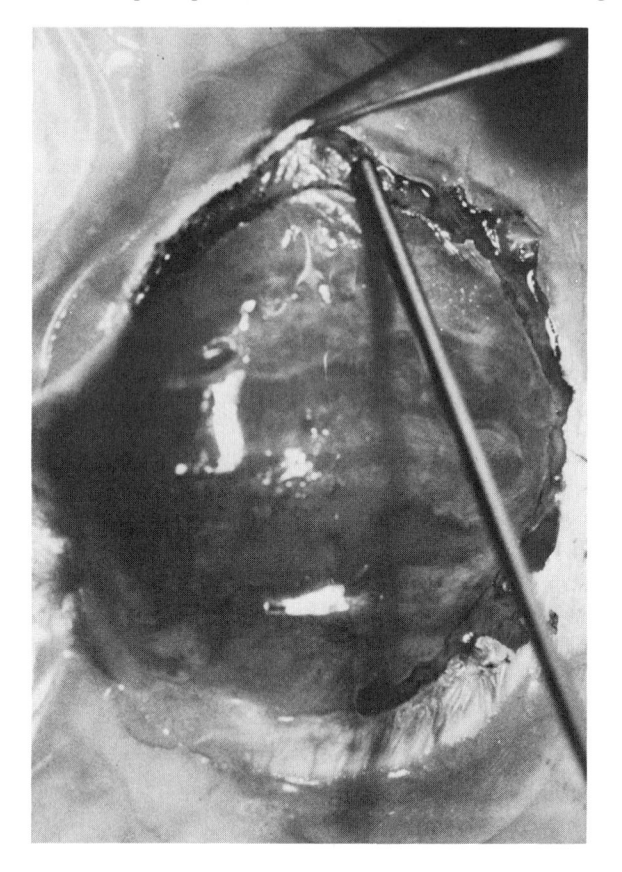

FIG 6–4.
Laser is used to incise the placode-skin junction. Note that at the tip of the instrument the subarachnoid space is still intact.

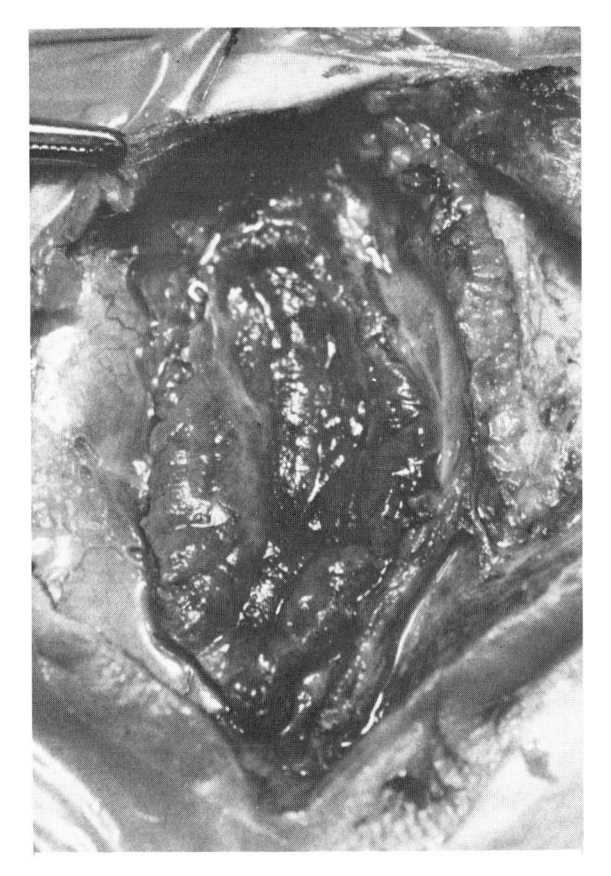

FIG 6–5.
The neural placode is totally free and falls into the spinal canal. The laser is then used to incise the dura mater at its junction with skin on the right upper quadrant.

laser is then used to open the ligamentum nuchae. The laser is a marvelous tool for this step. The loose connective tissue melts away under the beam, leaving a clean plane down to the posterior spinous processes and squamous occiput. The muscle and ligamentous attachments can then be cleaned from the arch of C-1 and the laminae of as many vertebrae as necessary to get below the vermian peg (Fig 6–7). Rongeurs are then used to remove the posterior portions of the vertebra. Bone removal should be limited to that portion of the lamina medial to the articular facets. Dura mater is then incised with a knife, exposing the cerebellar tissue. If the fourth ventricle is dilated on MRI (Fig 6–8), the laser is used to incise and remove a part of the vermian peg to open and drain the fourth ventricle (Fig 6–9). A dural graft is used to enlarge the space around the rhombencephalon elements in the canal.

SYRINGOHYDROMYELIA. — There is some confusion over the terminology used to describe the distention of the spinal cord by a fluid-filled cavity within cord substance. For the purpose of this discussion hydromyelia will be restricted to distention of the central canal of the spinal cord and syringomyelia to a fluid-filled cavity within the cord tissue. Both conditions can and often do exist together. However, in the vast majority of pediatric cases, hydromyelia is the problem.

Treatment is directed at preventing CSF from entering the central canal or allowing CSF to escape from the cavity. The exposure of the spinal cord is essentially the same as mentioned earlier. The laser is then used to fenestrate

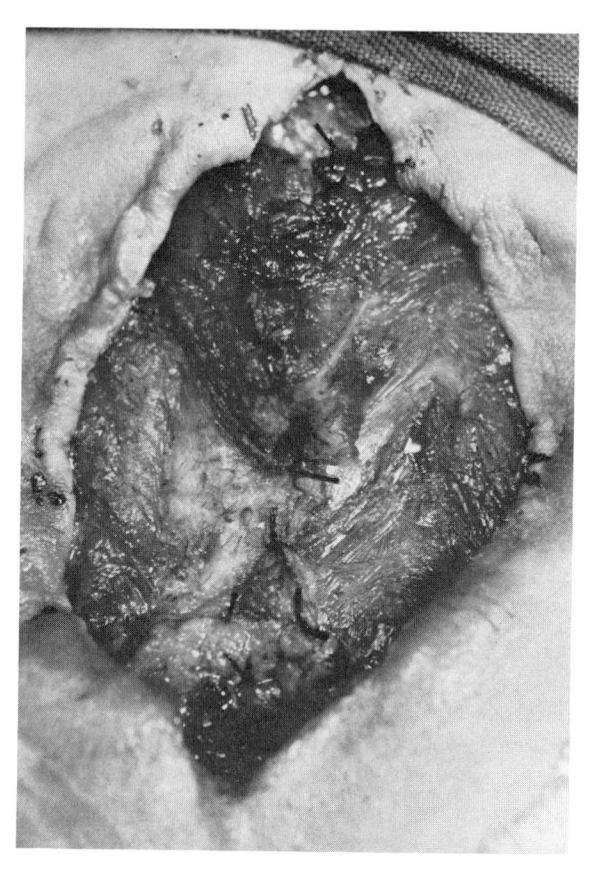

FIG 6–6.
Myofascial flaps are turned over the repair and closed in the midline.

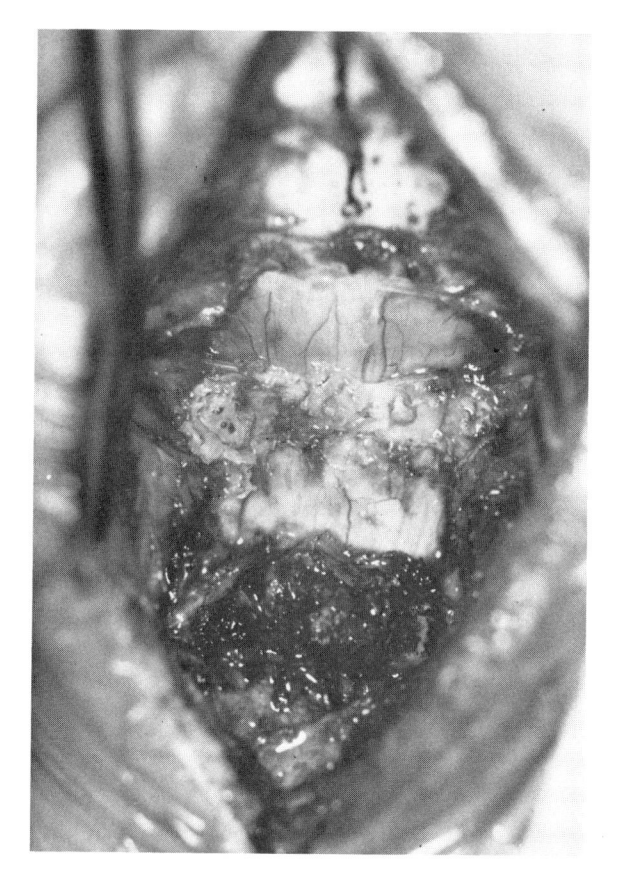

FIG 6–7.
This exposure was done totally with the laser. Rongeurs were then used to remove the posterior arch of C-1. Note how epidural fat can be simply vaporized to expose a clear dural surface. Also note the thick fibrous band usually present deep to the arch of C-1.

the spinal cord. The fenestration in children with a myelomeningocele and loss of sacral sensation is made in the midline. In other children, the fenestration is made in line with the dorsal root entry zone between dorsal roots. Again, magnification and low wattage are used.

SPINAL CORD NEOPLASMS. — Spinal cord tumors are not rare in children.[11] Most of the intramedullary neoplasms fortunately are benign. Recently, the large astrocytomas of the spine have been shown to be resectable.[6,7] The laser is particularly useful in removing the intramedullary tumors but also has advantages in epidural and intradural extramedullary tumors.

The approach to the spinal canal is essentially as mentioned in the previous sections. Intramedullary tumors are removed in the same fashion as intramedullary lipomas. A dorsal myelotomy allows the cord to be opened. Pial sutures are useful to evert the cord and expose the tumor. The laser is then used to vaporize the tumor, initially rapidly and then slowly at low wattage as the tumor-cord interface is exposed.

Using this laser technique, surgeons can accomplish gross total resection of large astrocytomas of the spinal cord without an increase in any neurologic deficits. In fact, most of these patients will have improvement in their neurologic examination results.

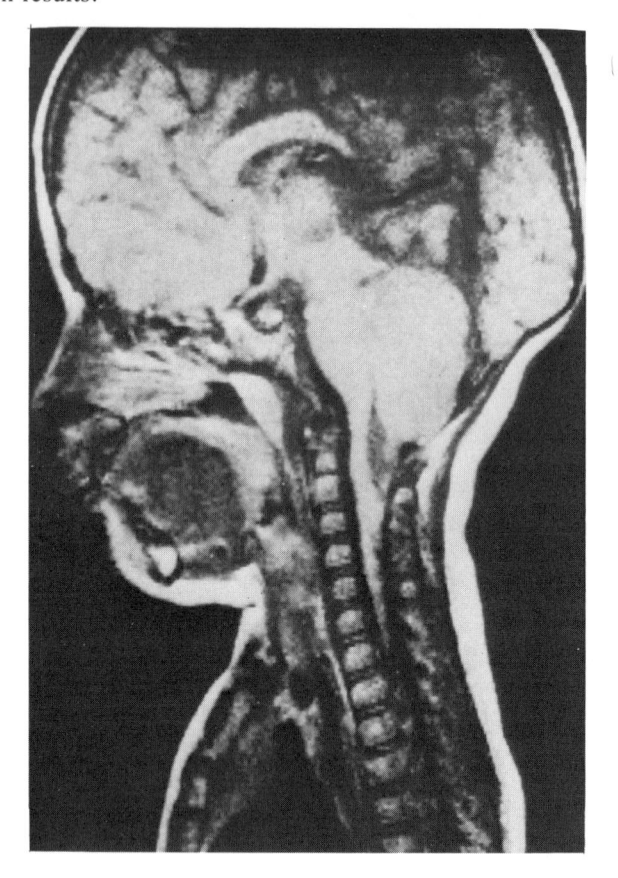

FIG 6–8.
A magnetic resonance imaging scan demonstrates the typical rhombencephalon malformation of the Arnold Chiari malformation. Note the low, dilated fourth ventricle.

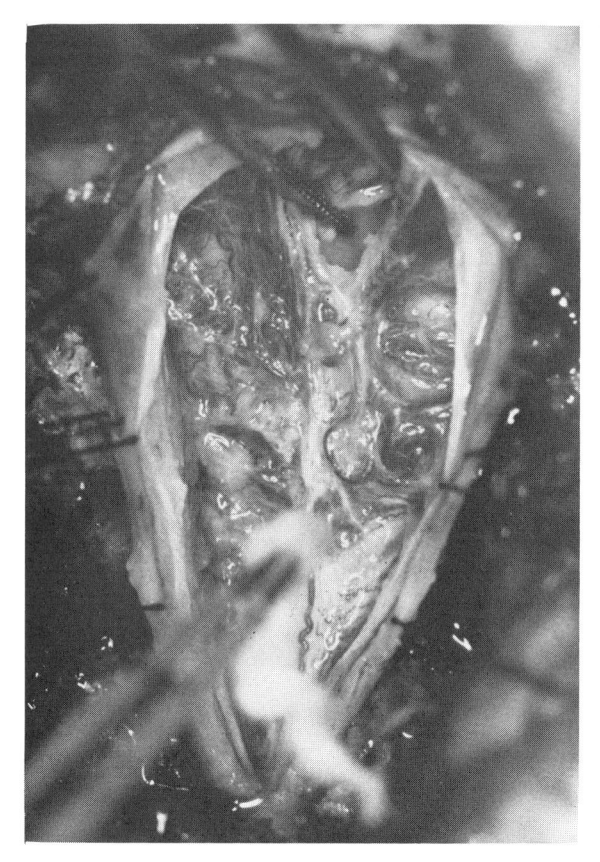

FIG 6-9.
The laser is used to incise the vermian peg to expose the fourth ventricle.

REFERENCES

1. Ascher, PW: The use of CO_2 laser in neurosurgery, in Kaplan (ed) *Laser Surgery II*. Jerusalem, Jerusalem Academic Press, 1978, pp 76–78.
2. Bruce DA, Schut L: Spinal lipomas in infancy and childhood. *Childs Brain* 1979; 5:192–203.
3. Boggan JE, Edwards MSB, Davis RL, et al: Comparison of the brain tissue response in rats to injury by argon and carbon dioxide lasers. *Neurosurgery* 1982; 11:609–616.
4. Burke LP, Rovin RA, Cerullo LJ, et al: YAG laser in neurosurgery, in Joffe (ed): *Nd:YAG Lasers in Medicine and Surgery*. New York, Elsevier North-Holland Inc, 1983.
5. Edwards MSB, Boggan JE: Argon laser surgery of pediatric neural neoplasms. *Childs Brain* 1984; 11:171–175.

6. Epstein F: Surgical treatment of extensive spinal cord astrocytomas of childhood. *Concepts Pediatr Neurosurg* 1983; 3:157–169.
7. Epstein F, Epstein N: Surgical treatment of spinal cord astrocytoma in children. *J Neurosurg* 1982; 57:685–689.
8. Epstein F, McCleary EL: Intrinsic brain stem tumors of childhood: Surgical indications. *J Neurosurg* 1986; 64:11–15.
9. Fernbach SK, McLone DG: Derangement of swallowing in children with myelomeningocele. *Pediatr Radiol* 1985; 15:311–314.
10. Fox JL, Stein MN, Hayes JR, et al: Effects of laser irradiation on the central nervous system: II. The intracranial explosion. *J Neurol Neurosurg Psychiatry* 1968; 31:43–49.
11. Gutierrez FA, Oi S, McLone DG: Intraspinal tumors in children: Clinical review, surgical results and follow-up in 51 cases. *Concepts Pediatr Neurosurg* 1983; 4:291–305.
12. Hendrick EB, Hoffman HJ, Humphreys RP: The tethered spinal cord. *Clin Neurosurg* 1983; 30:457–463.
13. Hoffman HJ, Becker L, Craven MA: A clinically and pathologically distinct group of benign brain stem gliomas. *Neurosurgery* 1980; 7:243–248.
14. Hoffman HJ, Stroink AR, Hendrick EB, et al: Pediatric brain stem gliomas in the CT era. *Concepts Pediatr Neurosurg,* in press.
15. Hoffman HJ, Taecholarn C, Hendrick EB, et al: Management of lipomyelomeningoceles. *J Neurosurg* 1985; 62:1–8.
16. McLaurin R: Hypothalamic gliomas in childhood. *Concepts Pediatr Neursurg,* in press.
17. McLone DG: Results of treatment of children born with a myelomeningocele. *Clin Neurosurg* 1983; 30:407–412.
18. McLone DG, Hayashida SF, Caldarelli M: Surgical resection of lipomyelomeningoceles in 18 asymptomatic infants. *J. Pediatr Neurosci* 1985; 12:239–242.
19. McLone DG, Dias L, Kaplan WE, et al: Concepts in the management of spina bifida. *Concepts Pediatr Neurosurg* 1985; 5:97–106.
20. McLone DG, Naidich TP: Laser resection of 50 spinal lipomas. *Neurosurgery* 1986; 18:611–615.
21. McLone DG, Mutluer S, Naidich TP: Lipomeningoceles of the conus medullaris. *Concepts Pediatr Neurosurg* 1983; 3:171–177.
22. McLone DG, Naidich TP: Spinal dysraphism: Experimental and clinical, in Holtzmann RNN, Stein BM (eds): *The Tethered Spinal Cord.* New York, Thieme-Stratton Inc., 1985; pp 14–28.
23. McLone DG, Naidich TP: Terminal myelocystocele. *Neurosurgery* 1985; 16:36–43.
24. McLone DG, Suwa J, Collins JA, et al: Neurulation: Biochemical and morphological studies on primary and secondary neural tube defects. *Concepts Pediatr Neurosurg* 1983; 4:15–29.
25. Naidich TP, Fernbach SK, McLone DG, et al: John Caffey Award: Sonography of the caudal spine and back: Congenital anomalies in children. *AJNR* 1984; 5:221–234.
26. Naidich TP, Harwood-Nash DC, McLone DG: Radiology of spinal dysraphism. *Clin Neurosurg* 1983; 30:341–365.
27. Naidich TP, McLone DG, Fulling KH: The Chairi II malformation: IV: The hindbrain deformity. *Neuroradiology* 1983; 25:179–197.
28. Naidich TP, McLone DG Harwood-Nash DC: Spinal dysraphism, in Newton TH,

Potts DG (eds): *Modern Neuroradiology: Computed Tomography of the Spine and Spinal Cord.* San Anselmo, Calif, Clavadel Press, 1983; pp 299–354.
29. Naidich TP, McLone DG, Mutluer S: A new understanding of dorsal dysraphism with lipoma (lipomyeloschisis): Radiological evaluation and surgical correction. *AJNR* 1983; 4:103–116.
30. Naidich TP, McLone DG, Shkolnik A, et al: Sonographic evaluation of caudal spine anomalies in children. *AJNR* 1983; 4:661–664.
31. Naidich TP, McLone DG: Ultrasonography versus computed tomography; in Holtzman RNN, Stein BM (eds): *The Tethered Spinal Cord.* New York, Thieme-Stratton Inc, 1985; pp 47–58.
32. Saunders ML, Young HF, Becker DP, et al: The use of the laser in neurological surgery. *Surg Neurol* 1980; 14:1–10.
33. Stellar S: Experimental studies with the carbon dioxide laser as a neurosurgical instrument. *Med Biol Eng* 1970; 8:549–558.
34. Tomita T, McLone DG: Acute respiratory arrest: A complication of malfunction of the shunt in children with myelomeningocele and Arnold-Chiari malformation: A report of three cases. *AJD* 1983; 137:142–144.
35. Tomita T, McLone DG: Posterior fossa ependymomas in childhood. Read before the annual meeting of the International Society for Pediatric Neurosurgery, Madrid, Sep 30 to Oct 3, 1986.
36. Walker ML: The use of the CO_2 laser for surgical treatment of intrinsic brain stem gliomas, in Hoffman HJ (ed):
37. Walker ML, Storrs BB: Lasers in pediatric neurosurgery. *Pediatr Neurosci* 1985; 12:23–30.
38. Walker ML, Storrs BB: Surgical therapy for intrinsic brain stem gliomas. *Concepts Pediatr Neurosurg*, 1985; 5:178–186.
39. Walker ML, Storrs BB, Goodman SG: Use of the CO_2 laser for surgical excision of primary brain tumors in children. *Concepts Pediatr Neurosurg* 1983; 3:297–315.
40. Yamada S, Zinke DE, Sanders D: Pathophysiology of tethered cord syndrome. *J Neurosurg* 1981; 54:494–503.

7 Glial Neoplasms: Conventional and Stereotactic Applications

PATRICK J. KELLY, M.D.

Intracranial glial neoplasms are the most common intracranial tumor in a neurosurgeon's practice. Approximately 12,000 Americans are afflicted with primary intracranial tumors each year, of which 80% are glial in origin; of these, 60% are malignant. Paradoxically, modern technology, including new imaging modalities, operating microscope, ultrasonic aspirator, laser, and improved methods of hemostasis, provides our patients no better long-term survival than did more primitive surgical methods practiced over 50 years ago.[18]

The first operation for glioma was performed by Bennett and Godlee in 1884.[1] They operated on a patient having a low-grade astrocytoma, but the patient died of infection. Harvey Cushing's philosophy on the surgical treatment of glial neoplasms evolved during his career. He first recommended a simple external decompression in which a biopsy specimen was obtained by craniotomy. Later, Cushing[5] advised radical "removal" of these tumors. The so-called internal decompression was popularized by MacKenzie for the management of high-grade glial tumors.

Jelsma and Bucy[11] reported that patients having radical resections of high-grade gliomas did better in the postoperative period and in long-term survival than did those having only a biopsy or partial excision. These tumors remain localized, grow by local extension, and metastasize only in very rare instances. However, they always recur locally and usually within a few centimeters of the site of resection, following even the most radical attempts at surgical excision.

More complete resection of glial neoplasms is limited, in part, by the surgeon's inability to accurately visualize the lesion as a complex, three-dimensional volume in space. Below the cortical surface, the boundaries between glial tumor and edematous white matter are not always clear. Surgeons, not wishing to inflict neurologic deficits, tend to be conservative in tumor removal, with the inevitable result that much of the neoplasm is left behind. In the case of high-grade gliomas, the average surgical decompression removes approximately 30% to 40% of the lesion. If one considers the growth rate of the lesion of up to 10% of its volume per week, standard internal decompression would theoretically slow the tumor's growth rate by only three or four weeks.

However, over the last 15 years, an explosion in technology has occurred. New instrumentation and imaging methodology have made possible new approaches for the study and treatment of intracranial glial neoplasms. Specifically, imaging modalities such as computed tomography (CT) and magnetic resonance imaging (MRI) can be used not only for the diagnosis of these lesions but also to define the tumor as a three-dimensional target volume in space. Stereotactic methods may then be employed for precise three-dimensional localization and aggressive resection of as much of the lesion as possible. Stereotactic serial biopsies based on CT, and more recently on MRI, provide new insights into the biology of these neoplasms.

To define better the histologic concomitants of CT- and MRI-defined abnormalities in intracranial lesions, we have performed over 600 CT-based and 125 MRI-based stereotactic biopsies on a variety of intracranial lesions, of which 305 have been primary glial neoplasms. We have derived the following conclusions based on our experience.

BIOLOGIC CHARACTERISTICS OF GLIAL NEOPLASMS

Individual glial neoplasms vary considerably in their rate of growth and the rapidity with which they invade normal parenchyma. Nevertheless, glial neoplasms have common general characteristics. Two major elements constitute most glial neoplasms: isolated tumor cells that invade intact parenchyma and solid tumor tissue.[7,13,14] Significant portions of most glial neoplasms consist of isolated tumor cells that invade the interstitial spaces into intact parenchyma. There, isolated tumor cells induce edema interstitially and intracellularly. Edema represents an increase in unstructured tissue water and results in low attenuation on CT scanning and in prolongation of both T1 and T2 on MRI. Isolated tumor cells are mobile and can travel great distances without destroying the basic structure of the brain.[2]

Some tumor cells are not quite as mobile. As these cells undergo mitoses, the local cellular population increases and the cells coalesce to form the other component of a glial neoplasm: tumor tissue. Tumor tissue induces neovascularization. Intense neovascularization is noted in higher-grade neoplasms; the extent of tumor is accurately reflected by contrast enhancement.[9,20] Furthermore, tumor tissue destroys underlying neural parenchyma, and tumor tissue thus has no viable parenchyma within.[3,6,8] High-grade glial neoplasms tend to undergo central necrosis, perhaps from outpacing their blood supply or from secreting toxic factors into themselves.

Serial CT scans on high-grade glial neoplasms demonstrate that the contrast-enhancing "ring" appears to grow as the zone of central low attenuation also enlarges, giving the impression that the lesion is growing by expansion.[3] Unfortunately this is rarely the case. These lesions grow by invasion and destruction of parenchyma. The isolated tumor cells in the infiltrated parenchyma increase in number, becoming coalescent, and form new solid tumor tissue that induces new neovascularity. The older tumor tissue elements in the central portion of the lesion undergo necrosis.

Low-grade astrocytomas result in a diffuse area of low attenuation on CT, occasionally with mass effect. Contrast enhancement is rare. Low-grade tumors

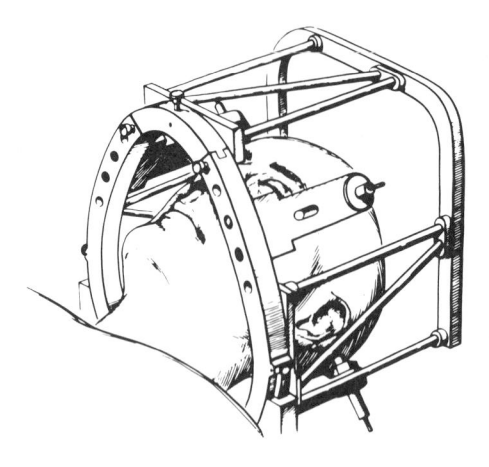

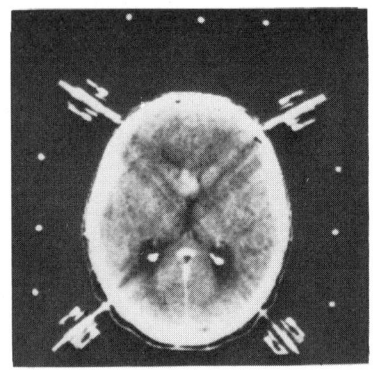

FIG 7–1.
Stereotactic computed tomographic (CT) scanning. Note nine reference marks around CT slice created by localization system.

also result in prolongation of T1 and T2 on the T1- and T2-weighted MRI images, respectively (Fig 7–1). On CT scanning, intermediate-grade neoplasms are characterized by areas of contrast enhancement within a low-attenuation field. High-grade tumors are manifest by contrast enhancement with a central zone of low attenuation. In both cases the T1 image on MRI usually demonstrates two or three different areas of T1 prolongation, whereas T2 is universally prolonged throughout the entire lesion. In all glial neoplasms the region defined by T2 prolongation is usually much larger than the abnormality indicated by CT scanning.

GOALS IN GLIOMA SURGERY

No surgical procedure has been proved to make a significant difference in the length of survival in patients with high-grade tumors.[18] However, selected lower-grade lesions can benefit from surgical resection. Significant prolongation of survival following surgical resection of low-grade lesions would be expected theoretically and has been demonstrated clinically.[16] Contemporary surgical philosophy for all gliomas includes three basic goals.

ESTABLISH TISSUE DIAGNOSIS

A tissue diagnosis must be obtained in all cases for selection of appropriate therapy and for prognostication. This has been traditionally achieved by means of craniotomy and open biopsy of superficially located lesions. With CT and, more recently, MRI-based stereotactic biopsy techniques available, there is little excuse for not establishing the histologic diagnosis in patients harboring deep-seated lesions as well as more superficially located lesions. Analysis of my own experience with stereotactic biopsies revealed that 17% of patients referred for histologic confirmation of their "tumor" were found to have nonneoplastic lesions.[12] The morbidity rate for stereotactic biopsies in my experience has been less than 1%.

INTERNAL DECOMPRESSION

Internal decompression is performed to reduce intracranial pressure and local pressure on vital structures. This is especially appropriate for patients whose tumors are composed of solid tumor tissue. A contrast-enhancing mass on CT can be removed with good postoperative neurologic results, as there should be no useful parenchyma within.[7]

REDUCE TUMOR BURDEN

Theoretically, chemotherapy and radiation therapy are more effective when less tumor burden exists. Unfortunately, major portions of glial neoplasms are frequently composed of intact parenchyma infiltrated by isolated tumor cells.[3,6,13] If the lesion is located in important brain tissue, postoperative neurologic deficit will always result from resection of infiltrated parenchyma.[14] Therefore, a significant reduction of tumor burden is only rarely achieved in glial neoplasms.

THE SURGICAL LASER IN GLIOMA SURGERY

Volume vaporization of tumor bulk would be an ideal application for the carbon dioxide (CO_2) laser in glioma surgery not provided by other means of tissue removal. Unfortunately, most commercially available laser units are hopelessly underpowered to vaporize significant amounts of tumor in an efficient manner. Thus, the CO_2 laser has only a few minor advantages over other means of cutting and tissue removal, including suction, bipolar forceps, and ultrasonic aspirator. First, it is relatively hemostatic. There is slightly less blood loss in removing a glioma with the laser than by more conventional means. Second, the thermal effects of the laser on the zone of neovascularization are useful in separating tumor tissue from infiltrated but intact brain parenchyma. The heat from the laser tends to shrink the neovascularized tumor tissue, which frequently develops a plane of cleavage between tumor tissue and infiltrated parenchyma. Third, laser incisions are more precise than those produced by conventional means. Even when 100 W of power is used, the thermal damage on either side of a laser incision rarely exceeds 300 μm.[19] This is especially important when resecting a glioma from important brain areas.

The CO_2 laser is convenient for removing tissue at the bottom of a deep cavity and is especially useful in resecting deep-seated tumors. Using the laser, these deep-seated lesions can be approached through relatively small cortical and subcortical white-matter openings. Only the laser beam and an aspirator need be in the surgical field during removal of the tumor. Furthermore, the laser can be directed from a stereotactic instrument for precision resection of deep-seated tumors.[12,14]

SURGICAL APPROACHES TO INTRACRANIAL GLIOMAS

The actual surgical approach utilized for the resection of a glioma depends on its location. At our institution, lesions located in frontal, temporal, or occipital poles are treated by lobectomy. Centrally and superficially located lesions are resected by stereotactic trephine craniotomy. Deep-seated periventricular, basal ganglia, and thalamic lesions are resected by computer-assisted stereotactic laser microsurgical techniques.

POLAR LESIONS

Frontal Lobe

Some gliomas may appear to be localized entirely in a frontal lobe on CT scanning. However, study of MRI frequently reveals areas of prolongation of T2 extending back into the basal ganglia and across the corpus callosum. Nevertheless, frontal lobectomy allows resection of the bulk of tumor tissue along with the infiltrated components of expendible frontal lobe.

Patients are premedicated with an anticonvulsant (phenytoin [Dilantin] and phenobarbital) and glucocorticoids (dexamethasone [Decadron]), 24 mg/day for two days before the procedure. With the patient under satisfactory general endotracheal anesthesia, the head is positioned on a headrest or in three-point fixation. A bicoronal skin incision is made behind the hairline. A frontal bone flap is developed between five burr holes positioned as follows: (1) superior-anterior temporal area below the pterion; (2) behind the coronal suture at its junction with the squamous suture; (3) ipsilateral to the midline anterior to the coronal suture; (4) ipsilateral to the midline between the coronal suture and the nasion; and (5) behind the zygomatic process of the frontal bone. The frontal sinus should be avoided in turning the bone flap. The size and location of the frontal sinus is noted on preoperative skull roentgenograms and as follows: the lights in the operating room are dimmed, the anesthesiologist places a penlight at the inner canthus of the ipsilateral eye, and the frontal sinus is thus illuminated through the skull and its limits are marked on the skull. The anterior inferomedial bone cut is then made in a fashion that will avoid the frontal sinus. After placing dural tack-up sutures, the dura is opened along the inferior and posterior margins of the flap, hinging it on the superior longitudinal sinus.

The lateral limits of the frontal lobectomy are marked with cottonoids on a line drawn for 1 cm anterior to the sphenoid ridge inferiorly to a point 1 cm anterior to the coronal suture. The cortical surface is coagulated with bipolar forceps and incised with a No.11 knife blade and scissors. The white-matter incision is deepened using a hand-held, slightly defocused (spot size 1 to 2 mm) CO_2 laser having 40 to 50 W of power. This will control most bleeding until larger vessels are encountered close to the undersurface of the pia.

The plane of the white-matter incision should be perpendicular to the surface of the brain. As the incision is deepened, the pial surface inferiorly and medially becomes apparent. The pial surface is coagulated with bipolar forceps and cut with scissors. Some of the medial subcortical white matter of the frontal lobe is removed with laser to decompress the medial hemisphere and allow it to fall away from the falx. The incision is then deepened medially toward the floor of the frontal fossa. Experience with the CO_2 laser will teach the surgeon that this instrument is best used for white-matter incisions. Laser incisions of the pial surface result in bothersome bleeding, requiring frequent changes of instrumentation to bipolar cautery and loss of time.

On the inferior medial surface of the frontal lobe, the olfactory nerve is separated from the gyrus rectus, and the cortical incision is then brought anterior to the olfactory trigone, thus preserving the olfactory nerve. Anterior frontal bridging veins are left intact until just before removing the specimen. Premature sacrifice of these will result in collapse of the frontal lobe and possible disorientation of the surgeon.

Occasionally during the course of the frontal lobectomy, tumor extension posteriorly is noted. In many cases, a plane of dissection can be developed between high-grade tumors and edematous white matter; thus, the posterior tumor extension is kept intact with the frontal lobectomy specimen. However, it is sometimes necessary to cut across tumor tissue in a frontal lobectomy, especially in the dominant hemisphere. In this case, remaining tumor tissue can then be vaporized with 40 to 80 W of defocused CO_2 laser power after removal of the lobectomy specimen.

The laser can be used to achieve hemostasis. Defocused low-power laser energy, having a power density of less than 10 W/sq cm, is useful for controlling the "ooze" of blood from cut tumor vessels. A watertight dural closure and, following replacement of the bone flap, a two-layer scalp closure are recommended.

TEMPORAL LOBE

These tumors are best treated by temporal lobectomy, especially in the nondominant hemisphere. The procedural aspects for a temporal lobectomy are as follows: The patient is positioned in the full lateral decubitus position and the head is rigidly fixed in three-point fixation. Two types of incision are satisfactory for temporal lobectomy. The so-called question mark incision beginning at the zygomatic arch following superiorly and posteriorly along the pinnae of the ear, then swinging superiorly and anteriorly to end just behind the hairline, gives good exposure of the anterior temporal lobe. This flap has been used in epilepsy surgery for years. Alternatively, a lateral horseshoe-shaped flap that begins at the zygomatic arch, swings superiorly and anteriorly to the superior temporal line, posteriorly to directly above the mastoid, and then inferiorly has the advantage in that it exposes only the temporal lobe. In glioma surgery it is best to utilize an osteoplastic flap, in which the temporal muscle remains attached to the bone plate. The muscle vascular supply may later prove important in these patients, who will be subjected to radiation therapy, chemotherapy, and long-term steroid therapy.

In a temporal lobectomy, the surgeon must access the anterior aspects and floor of the temporal fossa. Therefore, after turning the bone flap, the dura is stripped away anteriorly and inferiorly, and a craniectomy is done with the ronguers to reach the floor of the temporal fossa and the greater wing of the sphenoid. Dural tack-up sutures are very important to prevent epidural bleeding from dripping into the craniotomy defect during the temporal lobectomy. The dura is opened in the shape of the letter *H* with its horizontal limb located just below the midpoint of the flap.

The anterior part of the sylvian fissure is identified at the petrous ridge. An incision in the superior temporal convolution will mark the superior extent of the temporal lobectomy; a vertical incision 7 cm behind the temporal pole will delineate the posterior extent of the temporal lobectomy on the right side. A posterior incision 5.5 cm behind the temporal pole is recommended for left temporal lobectomy to avoid speech complications.

The cortical incision may be made utilizing the hand-held and defocused laser beginning at very low power densities to coagulate the pial vessels and then progressively increasing to higher power densities to incise the cortex. Unfortunately, this takes time. After the novelty of laser-made cortical incisions has worn off, most busy surgeons revert to bipolar forceps, knife, and scissors for making the cortical incisions. However, the laser may be used for deepening the subpial white-matter incisions as described in the frontal lobectomy procedure.

The plane of the superior incision should be directed toward the tentorial insucira. We utilize 50 to 60 W of defocused CO_2 laser power (spot size, 1 to 2 mm). Maintenance of surgical orientation is very important. Extension of this subpial incision superiorly risks entering the sylvian fissure and damaging sylvian vessels with the laser.

As the incisions approach pial surfaces, cortical bleeding will be noted, and it is best to retire the laser and make the pial incisions with bipolar forceps, suction, and scissors. As the anterior incision is deepened subpially, the pia of the anterior superior temporal lobe is coagulated with bipolar forceps and cut with scissors. Eventually the anterior incision can follow the tentorial insucira posteriorly and join the depths of the superior incision, which exposes the inferior medial aspect of the temporal lobe. The posterior incision is also deepened, and exposes the pia on the inferior surface of the temporal lobe, which is coagulated with bipolar forceps and cut with scissors. Eventually the inferior and superior incisions meet and the temporal lobe is thus isolated. The temporal bridging veins are then coagulated with bipolar forceps and cut. As in the frontal lobectomy, it is wise to leave these intact until the specimen is to be retrieved to avoid collapse of the temporal lobe.

Occasionally the mesial temporal structures are involved by tumor. The temporal horn is exposed by the incisions in the temporal lobectomy procedure outlined above. The uncus, amygdala, and parahippocampal gyrus can be removed up to the sublenticular portion of the internal capsule as follows: the temporal horn is entered, the hippocampus is retracted inferiorly, and the choroidal fissure is opened using microsurgical techniques. An anterior incision is deepened into the amygdala, and the amygdala is removed with subpial suction. An incision across the uncus is made with bipolar forceps and scissors. Care must be taken not to injure the anterior choroidal artery, which courses around the uncus and supplies the choroid plexus of the temporal horn. Injury to this vessel has a high risk of producing hemiparesis. Following removal of the temporal lobe, meticulous hemostasis, watertight dural closure, fixation of the bone plate, and double-layer scalp closure are performed.

Occipital Lobe

Tumors of the occipital pole in patients already having a homonymous field defect can be treated by occipital lobectomy. An occipital lobectomy must be done with extreme caution in the dominant hemisphere, since the risk of postoperative dyslexia in addition to the homonymous field defect is high. The skin flap for this operation is horseshoe shaped and based inferiorly, extending to the midline. Three burr holes are made, two located 1 cm ipsilateral to the midline just above the inion and 8 cm above the inion, and the third located above the lateral sinus and mastoid. Intermediate burr holes are recommended in older patients, where the risk of tearing the dura is higher. Care must be taken in removing the bone flap as arachnoid granulations are frequently located near the superior longitudinal sinus and bleed profusely. The dura is opened in the shape of an X. One of the triangles is hinged at the superior longitudinal sinus and hinged inferiorly along the lateral sinus. The line of cortical resection extends from the temporo-occipital notch inferiorly to the position of the parieto-occipital fissure superiorly. As with the frontal and temporal lobectomy, the lateral incision is deepened until the medial and inferior pial surface is visualized, coagulated, and cut. A handheld defocused laser can be used to deepen the subcortical incision.

CENTRALLY LOCATED SUPERFICIAL LESIONS

Conventional craniotomy, cortical incision, and internal decompression of high-grade gliomas has been the traditional method for the extirpation of centrally located subcortical lesions. However, a stereotactically guided craniotomy in which a small trephine craniotomy is centered precisely over the neoplasm offers several advantages. When the dura is opened in standard, large-flap craniotomies for centrally located glial neoplasms, the brain in a patient with a glioma is usually tight. Brain tissue protrudes out of the dural opening until most of the tumor has been decompressed. It is hard to believe that this previously intact but herniated brain tissue remains viable after such an insult. However, with standard neurosurgery, flaps larger than necessary are required to locate and deal with all extensions of the neoplasm. In addition, it may occasionally be difficult to find the lesion, and the surgeon embarks on a "search and destroy" mission.

Stereotactic control is used to center a trephine craniotomy directly over the stereotactically located lesion. The trephine need be no larger than the cross-sectional area of the lesion that is defined by CT contrast enhancement. Once begun, the actual surgical procedure requires less operating time than standard craniotomies, and the amount of tumor resected is much greater than in the traditional internal decompression procedure. However, stereotactic craniotomy requires new instrumentation and time for data acquisition and surgical planning.

Data Acquisition

A CT/MRI-compatible stereotactic head frame is placed on the patient's head and secured by carbon fiber pins inserted into 1/8-in. twist-drill holes through the outer table of the skull into the diploë. For frame reattachment, detachable micrometers are utilized as a mechanism for replacing the frame for subsequent data acquisition or surgical procedures.[13] Following frame application, the patient undergoes stereotactic CT, MRI, and digital angiographic examinations as follows.

A CT table adaptation plate receives the stereotactic head-holder. A CT-localization system, which consists of nine carbon fiber localization rods arranged in the shape of the letter *N* located on either side of the head and anteriorly creates nine reference marks on each CT slice.[12,13,15] Stereotactic CT scanning is done on a CT scanning unit (General Electric 8800 or 9800) gathering 5-mm slices through the lesion, utilizing a medium body format (see Fig 7–1). In some patients, stereotactic MRI information will also be useful.

The MRI-compatible stereotactic head holder is similar to that described for CT, except it is constructed entirely of carbon fiber and molybdenum disulfate and has no metal parts. The MRI localization system consists of capillary tubes

filled with copper sulfate solution, which also creates nine referen
each MRI image.

Stereotactic digital angiography (DA) is useful for localizing import
vessels that must be preserved and for localizing important sulci. A ta
aptation plate receives the stereotactic head holder on the DA units (G
Electric DF 3000 or 5000). A DA localization system consists of plastic (Lucite)
plates that contain nine radiopaque reference marks and are located on either
side of the head anteriorly and posteriorly. These create 18 reference marks on
each anteroposterior (AP) and lateral DA image. Digital angiography is performed utilizing a femoral catherization technique orthogonal and six degrees
oblique. Arterial and venous phases are obtained.

SURGICAL PLANNING

Following data acquisition, the achieved data tapes from the CT, MRI, and
DA examinations are read into the operating-room computer system (Data General Eclipse S140 [128K ram access memory, 192 megabytes disk storage]).
The surgeon views each of the CT slices and MRI images that demonstrate the
image and digitizes them as follows. The nine reference marks on each CT slice
and MRI image are detected automatically by an intensity detection algorithm.
This suspends the position of each slice in a three-dimensional computer image-storage matrix. Utilizing cursor and trackball, the surgeon traces around the
outline of the lesion defined by CT, contrast enhancement, and hypodensity,
and on MRI the definition of the lesion by the T1- and T2-weighted signal
abnormalities. Each of these digitized contours is suspended in a separate storage
matrix. A computer program then interpolates the intermediate slices at 1-mm
intervals between the digitized contours and creates separate volumes in space
by filling in each of these slices with 1-mm cubic voxels.[15] Thus, volumes
defined by CT contrast enhancement, CT low attenuation, and T1 and T2 signal
abnormalities on MRI are each established in the computer matrix. Each volume
assigned an identifying gray level may be displayed individually or all may be
displayed together on a computer display monitor. The stereotactic surgical
approach to the lesion is then planned, taking its three-dimensional shape and
important overlying cortical structures into account. The actual surgical approach
is expressed in stereotactic frame adjustments, which access a selected point
within the interpolated tumor volumes. The volumes are sliced perpendicular to
the intended surgical approach angles: collar; (angle from horizontal plane) arc
(angle from the vertical plane); frame adjustments provide the desired approach
trajectory.

SURGICAL PROCEDURES

The technical aspects of the surgical procedure will depend on whether the lesion is located superficially or deep. In the approach to superficial lesions, the stereotactic instrument (modified Todd Wells stereotactic frame) is used to center the trephine over the tumor. The relationships between the computer display of the circular trephine and slices from the CT- and/or MRI-defined tumor volumes, cut perpendicular to the approach angles, will orient the surgeon during dissection around and removal of the neoplasm. Deep tumors are removed with a stereotactically directed and computer-monitored CO_2 laser.

The patient is placed under general endotracheal anesthesia. The stereotactic head frame is replaced using the same pin holes in the skull, pin placements, and frame micrometer settings utilized during the data acquisition phase. The patient is then positioned in the stereotactic frame. The patient may be placed in any rotation in the stereotactic head frame that will provide a comfortable working situation for the surgeon. The computer makes frame adjustments to account for this rotation. After preparing and draping the head, the stereotactic arc quadrant is positioned. The selected arc and collar approach angles are set on the instrument. Through a stab wound in the scalp, a pilot hole is drilled in the outer table of the skull by a stereotaxically directed 1/8-in. drill. The scalp is then opened by a linear incision. A craniotomy is performed using a power trephine centered on the pilot hole. The size of the trephine selected is equal to or slightly larger than the largest cross-sectional area of the tumor viewed from the selected surgical approach angles that have been determined during the planning phase.

The computer displays the configuration of the trephine in relationship to the reformatted tumor outlines (Fig 7–2). This will keep the surgeon oriented during removal of the tumor. A section of cortex having the same size and configuration of the most superficial tumor slice is removed with bipolar forceps and scissors. We have found that cortex is nonviable when tumors extend to within 1 cm of the surface. A plane is then developed around the tumor utilizing a hand-held CO_2 laser or bipolar forceps. In addition, a stereotactic laser directed from a computer-monitored microslad mounted on the stereotactic arc quadrant may also be used.

The surgeon frequently refers to the computer monitor to visualize the configuration of the lesion at each successive slice during the resection as the lesion is isolated from the surrounding edematous brain tissue. The interior of the lesion should not be entered until late in the procedure. In this manner, a high-grade glioma can be removed as an intact specimen. A plane of dissection is *always* found around these tumors that corresponds to the contrast-enhancing margin on CT scanning. After the specimen has been removed, the "tumor bed" appears to be edematous white matter. Unfortunately, biopsies disclose isolated tumor cells within this edematous white matter.

DEEP TUMORS

The stereotactic laser approach to periventricular, basal ganglia, or thalamic tumors requires custom instrumentation, which includes a computer-monitored stereotactic frame, stereotactic retractors, extra-long bipolar forceps, and dissecting instruments. The stereotactic frame consists of a servo controlled three-dimensional motor slide system that positions the patient's head in the center of the stereotactic arc quadrant (Fig 7–3). Frame positions are recorded by optical encoders. Frame movements are activated by a control console in response to stereotactic coordinates generated by the computer. An operating microscope and CO_2 laser microslad are run on a motorized carriage suspended perpendicular to the tangent of a 400-mm arc quadrant. This slides into position when stereotactic control is required. The CO_2 laser beam is delivered to the microslad

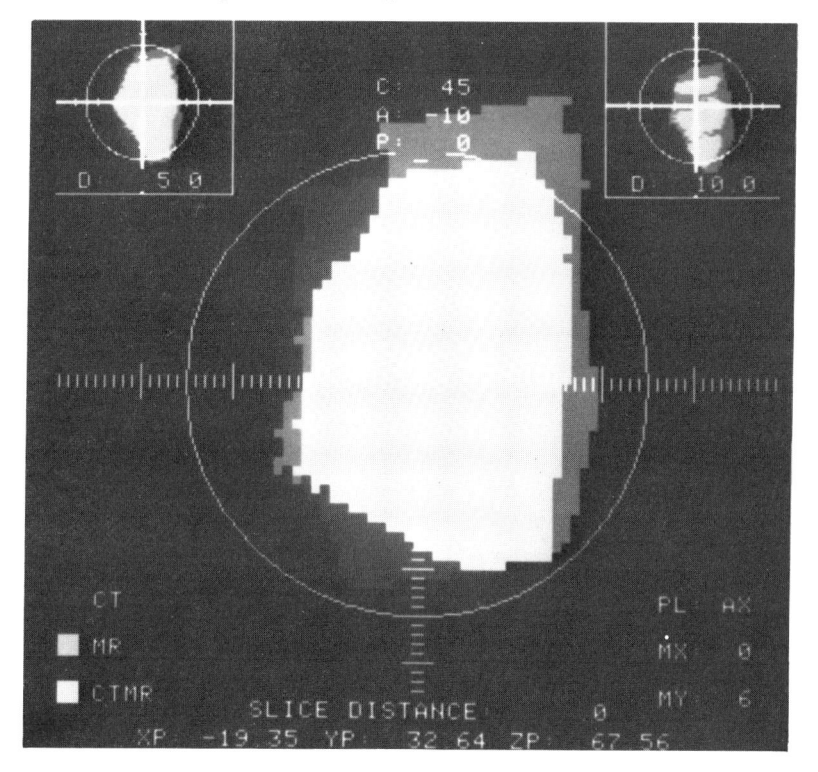

FIG 7–2.
Computer slices the computed tomographic (CT)– and magnetic resonance imaging (MRI)–defined lesion volumes in a plane perpendicular to the surgical approach. The CT– and MRI–defined limits are displayed as separate gray levels in relationship to the 5-cm-diameter trephine (*circle*) at a specified stereotactic level (*slice distance: .0*). A "look ahead" sequence demonstrates the configuration of deeper slices of the tumor (*top left and right of the figure*).

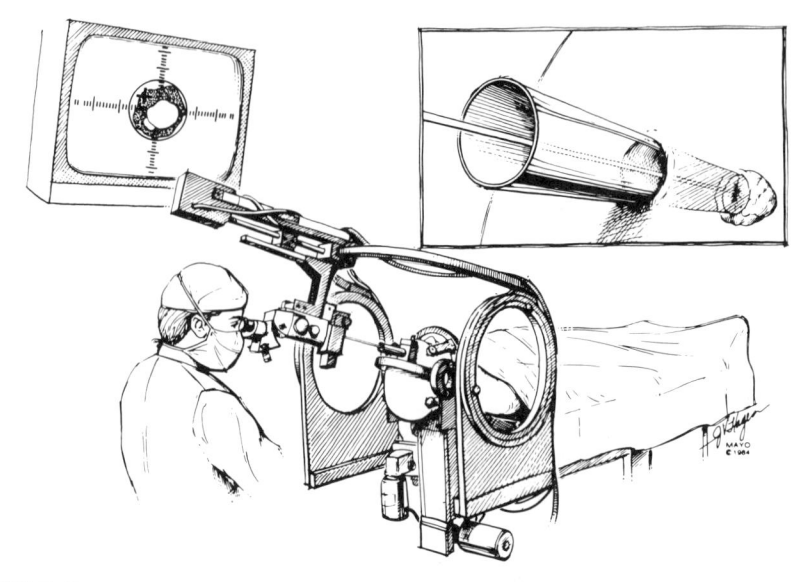

FIG 7–3.
Sterotaxic arc quadrant consisting of three-dimensional slide, 400-mm arc quadrant, and stereotaxically directed laser and retractor mounted on internal arc quadrant. Computer monitor displays reformatted tumor slices with respect to cylindrical retractor.

by an articulated optical arm. In the microslad, the laser beam is reflected by mirrors whose pitch is controlled by X and Y galvanometers, which direct the laser beam to the focal point of the arc quadrant. The mirrors are controlled by supplying precise voltage levels to the X and Y galvanometers, through the digital-to-analog output of the operating-room computer system.

The surgeon can move the laser to any selected position by moving a joystick that, through optical encoders, transmits that information to the computer, which in turn calculates and puts out the proper voltages for the microslad's galvanometers. In addition, the computer also displays the position of the laser (cursor) against a calibrated grid on a display monitor. The grid corresponds to the surgical field at the focal point of the stereotaxic frame. Slices of the CT- and MRI-defined tumor volumes cut perpendicular to the surgical view line (defined by arc and collar frame settings) are also displayed on that grid.

An internal arc quadrant holds stereotaxic surgical retractors. The position of these retractors is also indicated on the computer display terminal in the operating room. The position of the cylindrical retractor is shown as a circle on the display monitor in relationship to the tumor slice. A "look ahead" option displays deep tumor slices along the view line to provide information on the expected configuration of the tumor as it will be encountered as the procedure progresses (Fig 7–4).

Computer-assisted sterotaxic laser neurosurgical procedures are done with the patient under general anesthesia. The patient is replaced in the stereotaxic head holder and positioned in the stereotaxic frame. The selected target point within the tumor volume is positioned into the focal point of the stereotaxic arc quadrant. To monitor possible movements of the tumor during the procedure, a series of 1/2-mm stainless steel reference balls are deposited at 5-mm intervals along the surgical viewline in the tumor by a stereotaxically directed biopsy cannula inserted through a 1/8-in. drill hole in the skull. Anteroposterior and lateral radiographs are obtained. The positions of these steel balls on subsequent radiographs serve as indicators of shifts in the position of the tumor that may occur following craniotomy, opening of the dura, and exposure of the lesion. If a shift is detected (this occurs rarely, in my experience), the position of the tumor is moved accordingly within the computer matrix so that subsequent displays will automatically reflect the new position of the tumor with respect to the stereotaxic frame, retractors, and surgical laser.

The scalp is opened with a linear incision. A 1 1/2-in. trephine craniotomy is performed and a cruciate opening of the dura accomplished. A linear incision

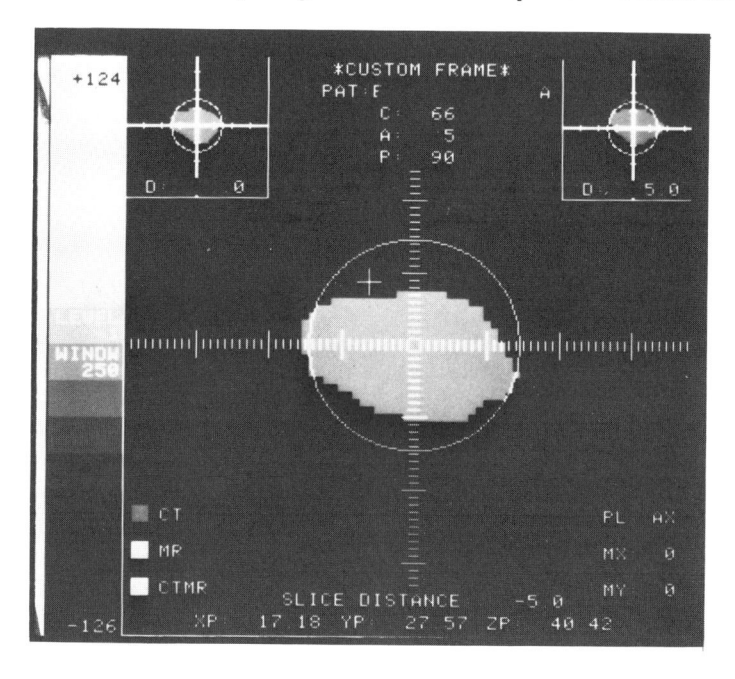

FIG 7–4.
Slices of tumor from computed tomographic– and magnetic resonance imaging–defined interpolated volume displayed perpendicular to surgical view line with reference to retractor (*circle*). Position of laser indicated by cursor.

is made in the cortex, and then the subcortical white-matter incision is progressively deepened with the stereotaxically directed CO_2 laser. The direction of the subcortical incision should be through nonessential brain tissue and in a direction parallel to major white-matter fibers. As the incision is deepened, the stereotaxic retractor is advanced to maintain the developing exposure.

The computer has calculated the range of the tumor along the surgical viewline. At the outer border of the tumor, the laser beam is deflected laterally and a dilator placed through the retractor, and the retractor is advanced. This creates a shaft from the surface to the outer border of the tumor. Using the computer display as a guide, the surgeon creates a plane of dissection around the lesion with the laser, advances the retractor, and deepens the incision circumscribing the tumor. Tumor tissue within the retractor is then removed with 65 to 85 W of defocused laser power utilizing manual or automatic mode (in which the computer sweeps the laser beam by specified programmed sequence based on the CT- or MRI-defined tumor limits). The tumor is removed slice by slice, extending from the most superficial slices to the deepest. Hemostasis is secured utilizing the extra-long bipolar forceps. The surgeon monitors not only the surgical field view through the operating microscope but also the display monitor for information on the location of the laser and retractor to the CT- and MRI-defined tumor boundaries. Anteroposterior and lateral teleradiographs are obtained to document the progress of the procedure and record possible movements of the reference balls (which are removed as they are encountered during the procedure).

Occasionally tumors larger than the retractor opening are encountered. In this situation, one side of the tumor is positioned under the retractor, and the surgeon separates this side from brain tissue. The display image is then translated on the computer display terminal to position the other side of the lesion under the retractor. The computer calculates new stereotaxic frame adjustments, which are duplicated on the frame by means of the control panel. This side is then separated from brain tissue with the laser. After isolating the lesion from surrounding brain tissue, it may then be vaporized by laser as described above.

Ultimately, a cavity is produced in the brain by removal of the lesion. This may be monitored by AP and lateral teleradiographs, and these may be compared with coronal and sagittal examinations of CT data through the tumor. The cavity produced should resemble the configuration of the tumor in location, shape, and size.

With these stereotaxic methods, it is possible to remove any portion or all of a lesion selected by the surgeon from CT scanning or MRI imaging. The procedure has been found to be most effective for the resection of circumscribed lesions from deep-seated intra-axial locations. For instance, pilocytic astrocytomas can be removed with minimal morbidity from any subcortical location,

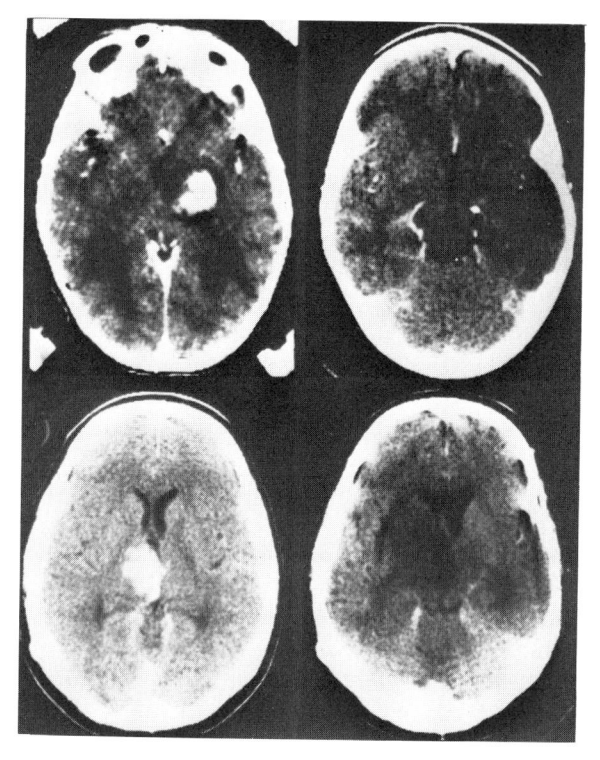

FIG 7-5.
Preoperative and postoperative computed tomographic scans in two patients having pilocytic astrocytomas resected from the left (*top*) and right (*bottom*) thalamus. Neither patient had postoperative deficit.

including the thalamus, by this method (Fig 7–5). These are circumscribed lesions with no infiltrating components.

With high-grade lesions, the tumor tissue component corresponds to the volume of tissue defined by contrast enhancement on CT scanning. However, lesions composed primarily of infiltrated parenchyma are not appropriate for this method when they involve important brain tissue. In low-grade lesions, the tumor tissue component is hypodense on CT scanning and indistinguishable from parenchyma infiltrated by tumor cells. The only method by which the limits of tumor tissue can be determined in these low-grade lesions is by serial stereotaxic biopsy, which is done as a separate procedure before computer-assisted stereotaxic laser craniotomy.

CONCLUSIONS

The surgeon must individualize the surgical approach and carefully consider the goals of what each procedure will accomplish in every patient harboring a glioma. Standard and stereotaxic surgical resection can only achieve two ends: to establish the diagnosis and to resect the solid tumor tissue components of the lesion. Therefore it is important first to establish that solid tumor tissue represents a significant portion of the patient's tumor. With high-grade lesions, the contrast-enhancing portion of the lesion on CT respresents tumor tissue. In low-grade lesions characterized by hypodensity on CT scanning, a stereotaxic serial biopsy is necessary to delineate tumor tissue from infiltrated parenchyma.[6,8,13]

Unfortunately, regardless of the technology employed for the removal of tumor tissue, these lesions will always recur because infiltrating tumor cells invade intact parenchyma, which cannot be resected if neurologic deficit is to be avoided.[3,4,13,14] At present, external beam radiation therapy and chemotherapy are the only generally accepted means of treating parenchyma infiltrated by isolated tumor cells. The problem is selectivity: we require a method that inflicts lethal damage to highly mobile and mitotically active tumor cells but that spares normal neural and glial elements.

Photoradiation therapy has been proposed. Here, a photodynamic drug is administered intravenously, incorporated by tumor cells and cleared from normal tissue.[10] Application of laser light of a proper wavelength to the tissue results in the formation of singlet oxygen and disruption of cell membranes in tumor cells that have incorporated the drug. However, we must solve problems relating to delivery of the drug to individual glial tumor cells and develop methods for the efficient administration of light energy to areas that may be far away from the surgically produced cavity following resection. Fiberoptic bundles stereotaxically implanted within the infiltrated tissue may be a viable means for delivering the proper wavelength light throughout the infiltrated tissue.

REFERENCES
1. Bennett H, Godlee RJ: Excision of a tumor from the brain. *Lancet* 1884; 2:1090–1091.
2. Brant-Zawadski M, David PL, Crooks LE, et al: NMR demonstration of cerebral abnormalities: Comparision with CT. *AJNR* 1983; 4:117–124.
3. Burger PC: Pathologic anatomy and CT correlations in the glioblastoma multiforme. *Appl Neurophysiol* 1983; 46:180–187.
4. Burger PC, Dubois PJ, Schold SC Jr. et al: Computerized tomographic and pathologic studies of the untreated, quiescent, and recurrent glioblastoma multiforme. *J Neurosurg* 1983; 59:159–168.
5. Cushing H: *Intracranial Tumors: Notes Upon a Series of 2,000 Verified Cases With Surgical-Mortality Percentages Pertaining Thereto.* Springfield, II, Charles C Thomas, Publisher, 1932.

6. Daumas-Duport C, Monsaingeon V, Szenthe L, et al: Serial stereotactic biopsies: A double histologic code of gliomas according to malignancy and 3-D configuration, as an aid to therapeutic decision and assessment of results. *Appl Neurophysiol* 1982; 45:431–437.
7. Daumas-Duport C, Monsaingeon V, N'Guyen JP, et al: Some correlations between histological and CT aspects of cerebral gliomas contributing to the choice of significant trajectories for stereotactic biopsies. *Acta Neurochir Suppl* 1984; 185–194.
8. Daumas-Duport C, Scheithauer BW, Kelly PJ: Spatial definition of gliomas by histologic and cytologic methods: Criteria for their application to stereotactic biopsies. *Mayo Clin Proc* 1987; 62:435–449.
9. Hochberg FH, Pruitt A: Assumptions in the radiotherapy of glioblastoma. *Neurology* 1980; 30:907–911.
10. Hoshino T: A commentary on the biology and growth kinetics of low-grade and high-grade gliomas. *J Neurosurg* 1984; 61:895–900.
11. Jelsma R, Bucy PC: The treatment of glioblastoma of the brain. *J Neurosurg* 1967; 27:388–400.
12. Kelly PJ: Computer-assisted stereotaxis: New approaches for the management of intracranial intra-axial tumors. *Neurology* 1986; 36:535–541.
13. Kelly PJ, Daumas-Duport C, Kispert DB, et al: Histological and volumetric analysis of untreated intracranial glial neoplasms studied by computed tomography and magnetic resonance imaging-based stereotactic serial biopsies. *J Neurosurg,* in press.
14. Kelly PJ, Kall BA, Goerss S, et al: Computer-assisted stereotaxic laser resection of intra-axial brain neoplasms. *J Neurosurg* 1986; 64:427–439.
15. Kelly PJ, Kall BA, Goerss SJ: Transposition of volumetric information derived from computed tomography scanning into stereotactic space. *Surg Neurol* 1984; 21:465–471.
16. Laws ER Jr, Taylor WF, Clifton MB, et al: Neurosurgical management of low-grade astrocytoma of the cerebral hemispheres. *J Neurosurg* 1984: 61:665–673.
17. Laws ER Jr, Cortese DA, Kinsey JH, et al: Photoradiation therapy in the treatment of malignant brain tumors: A phase I (feasibility) study. *Neurosurgery* 1981; 9:672–678.
18. Salcman M: Survival in glioblastoma: Historical perspective. *Neurosurgery* 1980; 7:435–439.
19. Stellar S, Polanyi TG, Bredemeir HC: Experimental studies with the carbon dioxide laser as a neurosurgical instrument. *Med Biol Eng Comput* 1970; 8:549–558.
20. Tchang S, Scotti G, Terbrugge K, et al: Computerized tomography as a possible aid to histological grading of supertentorial gliomas. *J Neurosurg* 1977; 46:735–739.

8 Intraspinal Tumors

JON H. ROBERTSON, M.D.

W. CRAIG CLARK, M.D., PH.D.

In adults, the ratio between intraspinal and intracranial tumors is roughly one to four.[37] Several excellent reviews concerning the epidemiology, pathology, and diagnosis of these lesions are available to the reader for further detail.[22,23,30,31,37,38] The purpose of this chapter is to discuss specific applications of laser technology in the operative management of various intraspinal lesions and present selected material to illustrate these applications. These tumors may be classified based on their relationship to the dura and the spinal cord. The distribution of intraspinal tumors by location and order of frequency includes (1) extradural, (2) intradural-extramedullary, and (3) intramedullary.

EXTRADURAL TUMORS

Approximately 30% of all intraspinal tumors are found in the epidural space.[37] Most epidural tumors in the spinal canal will be metastatic in origin, arising from a vertebral body and invading the anterior epidural space.[35] The most common sites of origin of these lesions are from carcinoma of the lung in men and carcinoma of the breast in women. Other primary tumor sites for metastasis include prostatic carcinoma, tumors of the gastrointestinal tract, thyroid carcinoma, and cells arising from tissue of reticuloendothelial origin.[37]

A surgical approach in suspected metastatic epidural carcinoma must be based on multiple factors, including (1) evidence of widespread metastasis, (2) age, (3) general health, and (4) preservation of neurologic function. In earlier reports that recommended immediate decompressive laminectomy, clinical improvement was seen in only 30% to 40% of patients.[2,13,16,29,43,45] Recent studies have suggested that the treatment of choice for most patients with metastatic cord compression should be radiation therapy rather than surgery.[5,14,18] A decompressive laminectomy with subtotal removal of epidural metastatic carcinoma should be performed only when (1) the nature of the primary tumor is not known or the diagnosis is in doubt; (2) relapse occurs following radiation therapy and no further radiation can be administered; or (3) symptoms progress despite ongoing radiation therapy.[42]

The anterior origin of most epidural metastatic masses makes a posterior decompressive laminectomy strictly palliative and diagnostic, since the majority of the compressive epidural metastatic tumor will not be visualized via a posterior approach.[8] If the vertebral body is already destroyed by tumor, removal of the posterior elements can result in segmental instability and further damage to an already compromised spinal cord.[44] On occasion, isolated metastatic involvement of a vertebral body with cord compression may call for an anterior surgical intervention[35,36] followed by a posterior approach for stabilization, if necessary. Following decompression of the epidural space, stabilization is usually performed if more than 50% of the width of the vertebral body has been removed or if the spine was rendered unstable by a previous laminectomy or tumorous involvement of the posterior elements[35]; it may be performed using instrumentation, bone grafting, cement, or some combination of these.[25,35,36] The reader is referred to several reviews examining the merits of these approaches,[1,6,26,35,36,40] as a complete exposition of these various operative strategies is beyond the scope of this chapter.

We have been unable to document any statistically significant difference in the outcome of patients operated on with the laser vs. those operated on with conventional technique when dealing with extradural metastatic carcinoma. The prognosis and result of any treatment strategy are functions of the general condition of the patient, extent of metastasis, and preoperative neurologic function. If a posterior decompressive laminectomy is performed for an epidural metastatic carcinoma, we would recommend standard instrumentation for biopsy and decompression, with coagulation provided by bipolar cautery. This approach is based on the following: (1) the tumor to be removed is visible posteriorly or laterally and can usually be stripped from the dura without difficulty; (2) coagulation in the epidural space is best achieved with bipolar cautery or application of gelatin sponges or absorbable fabric (Gelfoam or Surgicel); and (3) the use of the laser only increases the anesthetic time in patients who are often poor surgical risks and frequently have abnormal clotting related to their underlying metastic disease.

In the selected case of an extradural tumor of benign origin, such as a ''dumbbell'' neurofibroma, the decision to use the carbon dioxide (CO_2) surgical laser should be based on the location of the tumor and consistency and vascularity of the tissue. The CO_2 laser would provide coagulation with cavitation of the mass, with mobilization accomplished with bipolar cautery and standard microsurgical technique.

INTRADURAL-EXTRAMEDULLARY TUMORS

The vast majority of tumors in this location are either meningiomas or neurinomas.[17,21,23,28,37] Both of these tumor types are encapsulated and benign and usually separate easily from the spinal cord. They are small, rounded tumors and only become symptomatic late in their course, as the result of very slow growth. Meningiomas are most often found in the thoracic region (81%), with far fewer located in the cervical (16%) or lumbar (3%) areas.[37] Neurinomas are fairly evenly distributed throughout the spine, with thoracic neurinomas accounting for 39% of the total, lumbar 32%, and cervical 23%.[21] Neurinomas occasionally present as dumbbell tumors both within and outside the spinal canal.[23]

Most subdural meningiomas are attached to the anterolateral wall of the dura, with only a few attached to the posterior wall.[23] When a meningioma is attached to the posterior or postero lateral wall of the dura, it is often possible to incise the dura around the tumor's attachment, achieve dural hemostasis with bipolar coagulation, and simply lift the tumor from its bed in the spinal cord. If the tumor capsule adheres to the cord or there is difficulty in identifying the dural attachment, the laser may be used to decompress the tumor mass internally and allow retraction only of the tumor itself rather than the spinal cord. In anterolateral meningiomas, the spinal cord appears displaced backward and to the opposite side, with the nerve roots and dentate ligaments stretched. The dentate ligaments are secured with a small suture for retraction and then sectioned. An effort should be made to preserve all nerve roots, but this is often very difficult to do. The spinal cord is then rotated gently by retracting the dentate ligaments with exposure of the tumor. When the tumor is large, and the space available insufficient, the operator may remove one or more articular facets on the side of the tumor to improve the exposure. The spinal cord and nerve roots should be protected with application of cotton pledgets or Gelfoam soaked in physiologic solution as the tumor is approached. For tumors located anterior to the spinal cord, the tumor should be approached using an anterior or anterolateral approach, as outlined earlier in the discussion of metastatic tumors. After removal of meningioma, a free graft of bank dura mater, synthetic dural substitute, or fascia lata is applied to the ventral surface of the spinal cord and folded back on the dorsal surface like a hammock in an attempt to prevent a cerebrospinal fluid leak.[23]

The indications for using the CO_2 surgical laser attached to the operating microscope in removing intraspinal meningiomas is based on (1) the location of the tumor in relationship to the spinal cord, (2) the vascularity of the tumor, and (3) the consistency of the mass. The laser is used to decompress the tumor mass internally without applying major distracting forces to the spinal cord. This general technique of cavitation is accomplished with a defocused beam of CO_2 laser in a range of 30 to 60 W. The level of energy used in the decompression is related to the size of the tumor mass and its consistency. Mobilization of the tumor capsule is accomplished with the bipolar cautery and microsurgical dissection. Dura involved by tumor is removed by the defocused CO_2 laser beam.

Neurinomas found within the dura are removed much like the meningiomas. The major difference is that removing meningiomas requires removal of the dural attachment, whereas in neurinomas it is often necessary to section the nerve roots from which the tumors arise if the tumor capsule cannot be isolated from the nerve roots.

Dumbbell neurinomas present a different set of technical problems. These tumors may present with their major bulk within the spinal canal and only a small growth involving the intervertebral foramen (i.e., the bottle neurinomas), or they may present with an accompanying paravertebral tumor mass connected by tumor extending through the foramen. The bottle neurinomas present no particular difficulty, since the portion of the tumor within the foramen can be delivered into the spinal canal once the intraspinal portion has been removed. If a paravertebral mass is small, additional bone removal may be required, but its removal does not present any unique problems. In dumbbell neurinomas with a large paravertebral component, we have preferred a combined, staged approach performed in cooperation with another specialty surgeon because of the increased risk for chest or abdominal complications in the postoperative period.

INTRAMEDULLARY

Intramedullary tumors are the least common of the intraspinal tumors, with the reported incidence ranging from 14% to 30%.[7,9,24,30,38] The most frequently encountered tumors are ependymomas and astrocytomas.[19,24,27,32,38] Ependymomas are seen most frequently in the region of the conus and the filum terminale, whereas astrocytomas occur more frequently in the cervical or cervicothoracic region. Other intramedullary tumor types are generally benign, with malignant tumors being rare.

With the exception of new hemostatic methods and microsurgical dissection, the basic surgical technique for removal of intramedullary tumors has changed little since Elsberg's description.[9] Currently, we advocate the principles of (1) adequate exposure; (2) gentle, minimal traction when necessary on the spinal cord proper; (3) bipolar coagulation as an aid in maintaining hemostasis; (4) maintenance of a clevage plane between the tumor and the spinal cord with the assistance of the operating microscope; and (5) use of the CO_2 laser for performing the myelotomy and internal decompression of the tumor mass (Fig 8–1).

A complete laminectomy at the level of the tumor provides a posterior exposure. The dura is opened widely and the spinal cord inspected for discoloration, abnormal vascularity, thinning of the spinal cord, or other signs suggesting an intramedullary neoplasm. Myelotomies are generally performed in the midline with occasional paramedian incisions made, depending on the location of the tumor mass. If an avascular area is not apparent in the selected line of incision, a low-wattage (6 to 12 W), partially defocused CO_2 laser beam may be used to produce an avascular line for incision. The CO_2 laser is then placed in sharp focus (spot size, 0.5 to 1 mm) with low wattage (5 to 10 W) and applied in a pulsed or continuous fashion for the performance of the myelotomy. This technique of performing the myelotomy does not require any manipulation of the spinal cord with instrumentation. The focused laser beam incises the cord with coagulation of pial and tumor vessels. Minimal thermal effect is appreciated without the trauma associated with the use of a scalpel or microscissors.

As the myelotomy proceeds over the area of tumor mass, the tumor frequently

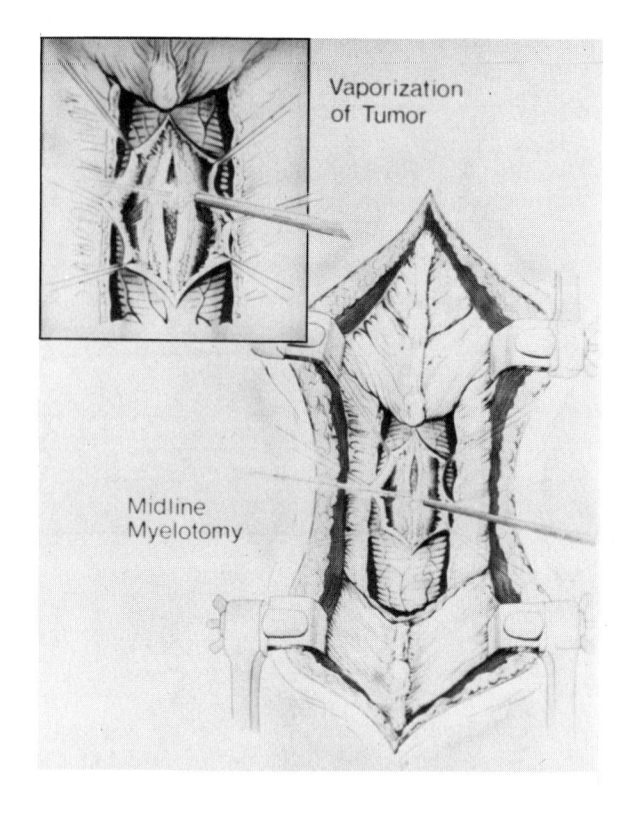

FIG 8–1.
Use of the carbon dioxide laser for performing myelotomy and internally decompressing the tumor mass.

becomes visible under the dorsal surface of the spinal cord. The coagulation effect of the laser easily divides vascular lesions that may exist between the spinal cord proper and the tumor mass entered. In patients who have had previous operations, adhesions and distortion of anatomy are frequently a problem. The cutting and coagulation effect of a sharply focused CO_2 laser provides a unique method for dividing pseudodura, adhesions, and vascular planes that may hinder the exposure of the tumor mass.

Tumor removal using the CO_2 laser consists of entering the mass of the exposed tumor, reducing the tumor mass via cavitation utilizing a higher-energy, defocused laser beam, and finally developing a cleavage plane between spinal cord and tumor mass with conventional microsurgical technique aided by bipolar cautery and continuous suction irrigation. Benign intramedullary tumor masses are easily managed with this technique. However, in the diffuse, infiltrating, low-grade astrocytomas or the more malignant intramedullary tumor masses, a

TABLE 8-1.
Surgical Laser Technique in Intramedullary Tumors

Myelotomy (cutting)
  Focused beam
  Pulsed or continuous wave
  5-10 W
Cavitation (coagulation-vaporization)
  Defocused beam
  Pulsed or continuous wave
  15-30 W

plane of dissection is often not easily appreciated, and one must accept a subtotal removal of tumor. The technique of progressive vaporization of tumor mass with a defocused, higher-energy (15 to 30 W) laser beam may be accomplished with a pulsed or continuous application of laser. The cavitation of tumor is accomplished with no mechanical manipulation or unnecessary retraction of the tumor mass or adjacent spinal cord.

The CO_2 laser has a very high coefficient of absorption and is absorbed by biologic tissues and converted to thermal energy directly proportional to the water content of the tissue. The thermal energy of laser light can be focused, and by varying the amount of energy and time of exposure, the effect on tissue can be precisely controlled. The method of application of the CO_2 laser for intramedullary tumor removal is summarized in Table 8-1. The operating microscope allows the surgeon to appreciate the effects of the laser on tumor tissue and facilitates a more precise attempt at tumor removal.

The surgical removal of an intramedullary spinal cord tumor is determined by the pathology of the lesion encountered. We recommend an aggressive surgical approach for removal of the benign intramedullary tumor; it is most effective in individuals who have minimal preoperative neurologic deficit. The diffuse infiltrating gliomas of the intramedullary space should be approached with the intention of total tumor removal. This has been reported by some authors[11,39] but technically may not be feasible.[20,24,30] It is emphasized that standard microsurgical dissection techniques are utilized in conjunction with the CO_2 laser. Bipolar cautery is preferred for coagulation of the penetrating vessels arising from the substance of the spinal cord entering the tumor capsule. Sharp division of these vessels is completed with microscissors. The bipolar cautery is also used in mobilizing the tumor capsule and developing the anatomic plane beween tumor capsule and the substance of the spinal cord. Continuous suction irrigation has been found to be useful in protecting against the thermal effect generated by bipolar cautery and laser.

UNUSUAL INTRASPINAL TUMORS

EXTRADURAL

The intraspinal chordoma is an unusual tumor that arises from a cell of origin in the spinal axis that ultimately differentiates into the cartilaginous component of the spinal canal. Arising from the vertebral bodies or sacrum, these tumors are slow growing and encapsulated and may be completely removed when accessible. The value of laser in removing this lesion is limited because of the tumor's avascular nature, soft consistency, and extradural location.

INTRADURAL

Angioblastomas and hemangiomas may occur as true neoplasms of the vascular structures of the spinal cord. Each of these tumors may present spontaneous internal hemorrhage in the substance of the spinal cord, with neurologic deterioration. They may be seen as part of a complex of vascular malformations associated with von Hippel-Lindau disease or Wyburn-Mason disease.

The CO_2 surgical laser has limited value in approaching these vascular lesions, and one might consider using either the argon or YAG laser. The bipolar cautery has been used effectively in removing these lesions with progressive coagulation of the arterial feeders and reduction of the tumor mass, followed by resection.

Epidermoid tumors and teratomas represent avascular, benign masses that may occur in the intramedullary space. An unusual avascular mass that is neither extramedullary nor intramedullary is the subdural lipoma. This unusually juxtamedullary subpial tumor is a lipomatous mass with a fibrous matrix having a fibrolipomatous attachment that arises from the tumor capsule and plunges into the nervous parenchyma.[3,12,15,34,41] Because of the lack of a sharp cleavage plane between tumor and nervous tissue, complete tumor removal has been considered impossible. A subtotal resection of the lipomatous mass followed by a dural graft to enlarge the intradural space has been the standard for managing this neoplasm. The CO_2 surgical laser has provided a new method for cavitating the subdural lipoma. This is performed easily as a result of the high water content of these tumors and the ability of the CO_2 laser to evaporate intracellular water.[4,33] The fibrolipomatous mass attached densely to the surface of the spinal cord may be completely removed to the level of the fibrous interface between the spinal cord proper and the lipomatous mass. Nerve roots that are densely adherent to the capsule of the lipoma are not disrupted. Tumor vaporization is accomplished with a defocused CO_2 laser applied in a continuous or pulsed fashion with a 20 to 40 W energy range. Because of the excellent decompression provided by the CO_2 laser without mechanical manipulation of the tumor mass, neurologic function is spared with no need for dural grafting.

The technique for removal of intraspinal tumors utilizing CO_2 surgical laser has been described. It is important that the laser be combined with microsurgical technique to achieve the full benefits of this technology.

REFERENCES
1. Ammirati M, Sundaresan N, Lane JM: Technique of vertebral body resection and stabilization for the treatment of spinal metastases. *Surg Rounds* 1985; 8:21–34.
2. Brice J, McKissock W: Surgical treatment of malignant extradural spinal tumors. *Br Med J* 1965; 1:1341–1344.
3. Caram PC, Scarcella G, Carton CA: Intradural lipomas of the spinal cord. *J Neurosurg* 1957; 14:28–42.
4. Clark WC, Robertson JH, Gardner G: Selective absorption and control of thermal effects: A comparison of the laser systems used in otology and neurology. *Otolaryngol Head Neck Surg* 1984; 92:73–79.
5. Cobb CA, Leavens ME, Eckles N: Indications for nonoperative treatment of spinal cord compression due to breast cancer. *J Neurosurg* 1977; 47:653–658.
6. Cook WA: Transthoracic vertebral surgery. *Ann Thorac Surg* 1971; 12:54–68.
7. DeSousa AL, Kalsbeck JE, Mealey JH, et al: Intraspinal tumors in children: A review of 81 cases. *J Neurosurg* 1979; 51:437–445.
8. Doppman JL, Girton M: Angiographic study of the effect of laminectomy in the presence of actute anterior epidural masses. *J Neurosurg* 1976; 45:195–202.
9. Elsberg CA: Tumors of the vertebral column, spinal cord and membranes, in Ellsberg, CA (ed): *Diagnosis and Treatment of Surgical Disease of the Spinal Cord and Its Membranes*. Philadelphia, WB Saunders Co., 1916, pp 236–281.
10. Elsberg CA, Beer E: The operability of intramedullary tumors of the spinal cord. *Am J Med Sci* 1911; 142:636–647.
11. Epstein F, Epstein N: Surgical treatment of spinal cord astrocytomas of childhood: A series of 19 patients. *J Neurosurg* 1982; 57:685–689.
12. Fromm H, von Wild K: Clinical aspects, operative treatment, and rehabilitation of paraplegia caused by lipomas of the spinal cord: With particular emphasis of the intramedullary lipomas. *Paraplegia* 1974; 12:15–20.
13. Giannotta SL, Kindt GW: Metastatic spinal cord tumors. *Clin Neurosurg* 1978; 25:495–503.
14. Gilbert RW, Kim JH, Posner JB: Epidural spinal cord compression from metastatic tumor: Diagnosis and treatment. *Ann Neurol* 1978; 3:40–51.
15. Giuffré R, Gambacorta D: Lipoma of the spinal cord. *J Neurosurg* 1971; 35:335–337.
16. Gorter K: Results of laminectomy in spinal cord compression due to tumors. *Acta Neurochir* 1978; 42:177–187.
17. Grant FC: Surgical experiences with extramedullary tumors of the spinal cord. *Ann Surg* 1948; 128:679–684.
18. Greenberg HS, Kim JH, Posner JB: Epidural spinal cord compression from metastatic tumor: Results with a new treatment protocol. *Ann Neurol* 1980; 8:361–366.
19. Greenwood J: Intramedullary tumors of the spinal cord: A follow-up study after surgical removal. *J Neurosurg* 1963; 20:665–668.
20. Greenwood J: Surgical removal of intramedullary tumors. *J Neurosurg* 1967; 26:276–282.

21. Greenwood J: Spinal cord tumors, in Youmans JR (ed): *Neurological Surgery*, Philadelphia, WB Saunders Co., 1973, pp 1514–1534.
22. Guidetti B: Intramedullary tumors of the spinal cord. *Acta Neurochir* 1967: 17:7–23.
23. Guidetti B: Removal of extramedullary benign spinal cord tumors, in Krayenbuhl H (ed): *Advances and Technical Standards in Neurosurgery*, New York, Springer-Verlag New York, 1974, vol. 1, pp 173–197.
24. Guidetti B, Mercuri S, Vagnozzi R: Long-term results of the surgical treatment of 129 intramedullary spinal gliomas. *J Neurosurg* 1981; 54:323–330.
25. Harrington KD: The use of methyl methacrylate for vertebral body replacement and anterior pathological fracture-dislocation of the spine due to metastatic malignant disease. *J Bone Joint Surg* 1981; 63-A-:36–46.
26. Johnson RM, Southwick WO: Surgical approaches to the spine, in Rothman RH; Simenone FA (eds): *The Spine*, Philadelphia, WB Saunders Co, 1975, pp 69–156.
27. Kopelson G, Linggood RM, Kleinman GM, et al: Management of intramedullary spinal cord tumors. *Radiology* 1980; 135:473–479.
28. Levy WJ, Bay J, Dohn D: Spinal cord meningioma. *J Neurosurg* 1982; 57:804–812.
29. Livingston KE, Perrin RG: The neurosurgical management of spinal metastases causing cord and cauda equina compression. *J Neurosurg* 1978; 49:839–843.
30. Malis LI: Intramedullary spinal cord tumors. *Clin Neurosurg* 1978; 25:512–539.
31. McGauley JL: Spine and spinal cord tumors, in Schneider RC, Kahn EA, Crosby EC, et al (ed) *Correlative Neurosurgery*, Springfield, Ill, Charles C Thomas Publisher; 1982, pp 975–1009.
32. Mork SJ, Loken AC: Ependymoma: A follow up of 101 cases. *Cancer* 1977; 40:907–915.
33. Robertson JH, Clark WC: Carbon dioxide laser in neurosurgery. *Contemp Neurosurg* 1983; 1–6.
34. Rogers HM, Long DM, Chou SN, et al: Lipomas of the spinal cord and cauda equina. *J Neurosurg* 1971; 34:349–354.
35. Siegal T, Siegal T, Robin G, et al: Anterior decompression of the spine for metastatic epidural cord compression: A promising avenue of therapy? *Ann Neurol* 1982; 11:28–34.
36. Siegal T, Tiqva P, Siegal T: Vertebral body resection for epidural compression by malignant tumors. *J Bone Joint Surg* 1985; 67-A-:375–382.
37. Simenone FA: Intraspinal neoplasms, in Rothman RH, Simenone FA (eds): *The Spine*, Philadelphia, WB Saunders Co, 1975, pp 823–836.
38. Sloof JL, Kernohan JW, MacCarty CS: *Primary Intramedullary Tumors of the Spinal Cord and Filum Terminale*, Philadelphia, WB Saunders Co, 1964, pp 3–9.
39. Stein BM: Surgery of intramedullary spinal cord tumors. *Clin Neurosurg* 1979: 26;529–542.
40. Sundaresan N, Galicich JH, Bains MS, et al: Vertebral body resection in the treatment of cancer involving the spine. *Cancer* 1984; 53:1393–1396.
41. Thomas JE, Miller RH: Lipomatous tumors of the spinal canal. *Mayo Clin Proc* 1973; 46:393–400.
42. Tomaszek DE, Mahaley MS: Management of spinal epidural metastases. *Contemp Neurosurg* 1983; 5:1–6.
43. White, WA, Patterson RH, Bergland RM: Role of surgery in the treatment of spinal cord compression by metastatic neoplasm. *Cancer* 1971; 27:558–561.

44. Winter RB, Moe JH, Wang JF: Congenital kyphosis: Its natural history and treatment as observed in a study of 130 patients. *J Bone Joint Surg* 1973; 55A:223–256.
45. Wright RL: Malignant tumors in the spinal extradural space: Results of surgical treatment. *Ann Surg* 1963; 157:227–231.

9 Vascular Applications: The Thermal Scale

CHARLES R. NEBLETT, M.D.

As neurosurgery has become progressively more refined and sophisticated, few anatomic areas have received greater attention than the intracranial and intraspinal vascular tree. This chapter deals with my research and concepts concerning the effects and, thus, the applicability of the microsurgical carbon dioxide (CO_2) laser.

THERMAL SCALE

Since the initiation of this research work in 1979, thermal parameters have received preferential consideration. Temperatures of less than 70°C result in an altered state of the exposed tissue. Biochemical and cellular changes may or may not be reversible, depending in part on factors of the exposure time and the temperature level.

At 70°C, fusion of organic tissue occurs. Thus, reconstruction of vascular tissue may be achieved. Only a few more degrees introduces the reparative effect. Vascular structures may be shrunk or sealed. A relatively unexplored area of approximately 20°C exists extending to the 100°C level. Destruction occurs at 100°C and above. Many changes and variances are observed at increasing levels. This scheme of thermal degrees will serve as the framework for this review.

ALTERED EFFECT

Little is known about this area in the thermal scale. At low levels of temperatures and time exposures, changes appear to be transient. However, as the time increases and/or the temperatures approach 70°C, the altered state passes from reversible to irreversible.

The exposure time and the thermal level have a complementary effect. Obviously, the shorter the time and the lower the temperature, the fewer tissue changes occur. Extended periods can be most detrimental. Extracellular water content in particular will be lost. The resultant "drying" of the tissues impairs their functional capacities. Extended, multiple, timed exposures can create this same undesirable effect more than prolonged continuous exposures can. Thus, it is desirable to lavage frequently the surgical field with physiologic saline solution.

Usually the biochemical and structural-cellular changes are reversible. As the temperature approaches 70°C, the effects are increased. When they are no longer reversible, interesting results can be noted. An example of this principle is seen in the border zone of the anastomosis site. This histologic work has been performed by Sharon Thomsen, M.D., of the University of Miami. The area of tissue bonding is within 100 μm of either side of the anastomosis in a 1-mm vessel. Adjacent cells may have irreversible changes occur. This results from the spot size being too large for the vessel, the application of the laser being sufficiently random to cause far-lateral exposure or thermal spread. A cellular dropout may occur, structural integrity may be diminished, and the healing will progress suboptimally.

Healing after fusion is significantly a migration of myointimal cells from the periphery into the divided portion of the vessel. These reparative cells then migrate from this position proximally and distally. However, the distance they can travel becomes limited, at least in part, by the septations in the remaining scaffolding of the elastic membrane.

Therefore, should the depopulation of cells extend for too great a distance, the healing process cannot be completed in those distal areas. A potential weakness may develop. Altered states offer a most interesting area for future research.

RECONSTRUCTED EFFECT

The reconstruction of organic tissue through applied microsurgical CO_2 laser techniques has generated a broad interest in the medical community. At about 70°C, the biochemistry of tightly apposed vascular walls is affected, resulting in a fusion of those issues (A. J. Welch, unpublished data,). At least in part, a protein denaturation-renaturation process appears to affect the tertiary amino acids, resulting in a thermal unlocking, then a reattachment, with the protein molecules bonded together. In-depth studies are essential to begin to establish more concretely the exact mechanisms.

The potential of organic tissue fusion initiated this entire research project. All research work has been performed in conjunction with James Morris of BioQuantum Technologies, Inc., Houston. The desire is to apply CO_2 laser forces in a microscopic mode with milliwatt and micron parameters to achieve this goal. The laser used for all of these studies is the BioQuantum Technologies microsurgical CO_2 laser model 7600.

The femoral artery of the rat is the basic experimental model. The artery is dissected free and cut transversely after microvascular clamps are applied. The artery is then reapproximated with three or four 10-0 microvascular sutures. The sutures provide firm approximation. Tension applied to two adjacent stay stitches facilitates the laser application to the anastomosis site. After each side has been laser fused, the microvascular clamps are removed and the anastomosis evaluated. Patency is established as well as its leak-free status. If bleeding does occur, then the opening is lavaged and refused.

Small or large, artery or vein, these structures can be laser anastomosed.

Several interesting factors should be reviewed. The wall thickness and the vessel diameter influence the laser values. The greater the thickness or the diameter, the higher the milliwatts that should be applied. A general rule of thumb is to multiply the number of millimeters in the diameter of the vessel by 100. That number is the approximate milliwatt level. For example, 1-mm artery requires 100 mW. Veins require less wattage because the walls are thinner. The chemical composition of the vessels varies, and therefore the milliwatts also vary. The microscopic mode and the microns are equally important.

The microscopic mode allows important visualization of the exact laser application and of the tissue changes associated with bonding. Precision is required. The more exacting is the exposure to the approximating edges, the more ideal are the tissue interactions. This will be more completely discussed during the consideration of microns. Second, the edges of the vessel are closely observed for visible tissue changes. A slight drying of the outer surface is noted, following by a darkening to a brown color. These alterations are difficult to perceive without the advantage of the microscope.

The spot size is measured in microns, not millimeters. The larger the spot size for a given milliwatt level, the lower the power density. To create the desired thermal effect, these two values must be considered. Also of great importance to this process is the length of lateral laser exposure beyond the exact anastomosis site. As described in the "altered effect" section of this chapter, the more the cells are exposed to the thermal force, the more likely is it that an undesirable irreversible change will occur. A structural weakness may result. Aneurysms may develop. Some alteration in spot size may be required when dealing with differing vessel-wall thicknesses and diameters. It is easy to remember, however, the important parameters of the laser for fusion, the three Ms: microscopic mode, milliwatts, and microns.

The success of the laser-assisted microvascular anastomosis depends on several factors. Experience and precision lead that list. We find that the success rate increases as we become more experienced. Also, the surgeon must pay close attention to several features, some of which may not be totally obvious.

Good apposition of the vessel walls is essential. Clamps are being developed to achieve this goal. In the meantime, approximating stay stitches are applied. Whether you choose to use three, as we routinely use, or four, as used by Dr. James Ausman, Henry Ford Hospital, Detroit, the tissues must be held firmly together.

There is no need to strip the adventitia. The adventitia may be fused over the media bonding, enhancing the quality of the anastomosis.

The time exposure varies with the surgeon. I prefer the continuous mode because there tends to be less drying of the tissues that may occur with multiple short exposures. Also, to prevent drying it is beneficial to bathe the surgical field frequently with saline solution.

Blood pigments should be thoroughly lavaged from the lumen and from the interface between the anastomotic surfaces. Thermally affected blood results in a "blood bond" that does not provide suitable structural integrity.

REPARATIVE EFFECT

In close proximity to the thermal forces that result in the reconstruction of tissue exists the reparative mode. Only a few additional degrees, or a few additional milliwatts, produce a shrinking and sealing response. This becomes important when applied to vascular anomalies.

Although the exact mechanisms remain unestablished, the effect on the collagen cells appears to play a role. The collagen cells become linearly aligned along the anastomotic site in the reconstructive mode.* This same type of alteration occurs with a change in collagen cell alignment from random to linear in the reparative mode. These cells also appear to thicken.

Two surgical applications are apparent, for aneurysms and for arteriovenous malformations (AVMs). Working at a microscope objective distance of 300 mm, with a spot size of 250μm and a power level of 100 to 150 mW, an aneurysm can be reduced in size. Should the neurosurgeon encounter an aneurysm that is difficult to adroitly control, this technique can be applied. Circumstances such as a giant aneurysm, poorly accessible neck, difficult angle for applying the clip, or excessive scarring may be facilitated by some shrinkage of the aneurysm. Microsurgical CO_2 laser application serves as an adjunct to the current armamentarium. It can be applied to a greater or lesser amount, as indicated.

In experimentally made aneurysms, the aneurysm can be shrunk with the laser in a reparative mode by increasing the temperature by an additional 25 to 50 mW, amputating the residual aneurysmal tissue, and sealing the junction between the neck of the aneurysm and the orifice of the parent artery. Although this has been successful, with good long-term healing, I have not performed this outside the laboratory.

The concept of shrinking, sealing, and ablating can also be applied to AVMs. The same parameters for the aneurysm, the three Ms, are used in this surgery. However, the milliwatts may be more rapidly increased. Obviously, the thermal force must be varied depending on the structural character of the AVM's walls, the amount and rapidity of blood flow, the adhesiveness of the arachnoid, etc. The objective is to shrink the vessels, arterial inflow first, and then seal them. When the malformation is completely sealed, then the temperature is increased from about 80°C to 100°C and the ablative mode provides cutting away of the malformation and its extirpation.

---

*Peter C: Lasers in neurosurgery. Read before the Texas Association of Neurological Surgeons, Houston, May 21, 1983.

The microsurgical CO_2 laser reparative technique may be used in conjunction with standard bipolar electrical technique or as the primary tool. Again, personal preference, experience, and varying qualities of the AVM all help dictate its application. Advantages include the "no-touch" and the "no-stick" qualities, as well as tissue effects that result and are somewhat different between electrical and laser techniques.

The reparative effect can provide benefits in other ways. For example, it is convenient to seal varicosities in spinal surgery. One advantage of having the microsurgical CO_2 laser always attached to the microscope is its immediate availability for use to reconstruct (as in "spot welding"), repair, or ablate.

ABLATIVE EFFECT

At 100°C water boils and cells vaporize. This is the spectrum of the laser scale most completely studied. It is this ablative area that has stimulated the application of lasers for surgery. This decade in laser neurosurgery has seen the evolution of its ablative use. Clinical indications have been explored; some are more applicable than others. New procedures are being defined; however, refinement may be even more important.

Precision of application with resultant enhancement of healing is the refinement being pursued. The no-touch technique is supplemented by the ability to "work the interface" between undesirable tissue and critical structures. A small spot size and a low wattage add finesse. They diminish the zone of destruction and reduce the amount of undesirable thermal spread.

Two temperature zones of interest for future development lie between 80°C and 100°C and significantly above 100°C, the "far zone." Other process applications surely will evolve from this new work.

CONCLUSION

This chapter has only superficially reviewed the thermal effects of the microsurgical CO_2 laser on vascular tissue. As we broaden our understanding of the resultant biochemical and structural changes, thermally induced, then the applications will increase and the refinements will occur for existing uses. For example, studies now in progress indicate that arterial fusion factors are as importantly affected by the biochemistry as by the size of the artery. In consort with these studies, investigations should be instituted to begin the understanding of the laser's nonthermal factors and the changes they produce.

10 Neuroablative Procedures

J. THOMAS BROWN, M.D.

Neuroablation involves the deliberate destruction of a small portion of the central or peripheral nervous system to attain a greater end. Although such procedures are not commonly performed, their results can be extremely gratifying, particularly when done in a quick, gentle, and precise fashion free of added neurologic deficit. The carbon dixoide (CO_2) laser, especially when linked to the operating microscope, theoretically provides the neurosurgeon with a precise instrument free of tissue manipulation with which to perform these rather delicate operations in a consistently safe and effective manner.

In this chapter, laser use will be described for two major neurosurgical problems. The first is the troublesome structural abnormality of syringohydromyelia, and the second is the surgical modulation of intractable pain due to neoplasia. It is believed that the physical properties and tissue interaction characteristics of the CO_2 laser render it an ideal instrument for such procedures. This is not meant to negate the usefulness of other currently available wavelengths but only to point out where most laboratory and clinical experience has been gained thus far.

SYRINGOHYDROMYELIA

Syringohydromyelia is a chronic progressive disorder characterized by muscular atrophy, dissociated anesthesia, paraparesis, scoliosis, neurogenic arthropathy, and other trophic changes.[1] The etiology of this cystic spinal cord cavitation includes congenital, degenerative, inflammatory, vascular, traumatic, and neoplastic mechanisms.[2] It is a disease process that is still poorly understood and, therefore, somewhat refractory to treatment. Problems with its surgical treatment include (1) the variable course of untreated syringohydromyelia, with the possibility of spontaneous arrest of the process[1]; (2) the many theories of pathogenesis that have evolved in an effort to provide a rational mode of surgical treatment[3-5] coupled with the probability that there is no single pathogenetic mechanism and, therefore, no one treatment method; and (3) the numerous methods of treatment with few long-term follow-up studies, making it difficult to determine which method is most effective.

According to Williams,[6] syringohydromyelia can be classified into a communicating type and a noncommunicating type, depending on whether or not the cystic cavity within the spinal cord communicates with normal spinal fluid pathways. Communicating syringohydromyelia can be associated with developmental anomalies of the rhombencephalon, such as a Chiari I malformation, or can be associated with acquired anomalies of the rhombencephalon, such as basilar arachnoiditis and posterior fossa cysts and tumors. Noncommunicating syringohydromyelia, on the other hand, is usually associated with spinal cord trauma, spinal arachnoiditis, or intramedullary spinal cord tumors.

Current treatment modalities for syringohydromyelia include (1) craniocervical decompression with opening of the foramen of Magendie and occlusion of the obex[3]; (2) terminal ventriculostomy at the filum terminale[7]; (3) syringostomy with or without a stint[8,9]; (4) ventricular shunt when hydrocephalus is present[10]; (5) syringoperitoneal shunt[11]; (6) cordectomy for posttraumatic syringomyelia[12]; and (7) laser fenestration with reconstruction of the meninges. The primary treatment objective, however, is to establish and maintain communication between the syrinx and functional cerebrospinal fluid (CSF) pathways. The CO_2 laser provides an ideal means to create a precise and theoretically permanent fenestration into the syrinx with minimal adjacent tissue damage and uninterrupted electrophysiologic spinal cord monitoring.

METHODS

The patient's diagnostic workup first includes roentgenograms of the skull and entire spine to determine whether or not associated bony anomalies are present. Iophendylate injection (Pantopaque) myelography (Fig 10–1), when done in both the prone and supine positions, can indicate both the presence and the type of syringohydromyelia.[13] This procedure, however, has largely been replaced more recently by metrizamide myelography combined with computed tomography (CT) of the spinal cord[14,15] (Figs 10–2 and 10–3) and, most recently, by magnetic resonance imaging[16,17] (Fig 10–4), both of which are usually diagnostic of the condition. All patients had precontrast- and postcontrast-infusion CT scans of the brain to rule out associated hydrocephalus and rhombencephalon anomalies. In addition to these radiographic studies, baseline somatosensory evoked potential (SSEP) studies were performed.

The surgical procedure consists first of a standard two-level bilateral laminectomy, preferably in the thoracic region. Intraoperative ultrasonography can be performed at this point to determine the precise location of the spinal cord cavitation and any asymmetry in the lesion (Figs 10–5 and 10–6). The dura mater is opened separate from the arachnoid in a crescentic fashion with the base of the flap anchored on the nondominant, usually left, side of the spinal cord. Exact hemostasis throughout the surgical opening is paramount to prevent blood from entering the subarachnoid space and possibly causing postoperative arachnoiditis and occlusion of the fenestration. The arachnoid is opened either with sharp microdissection or with the CO_2 laser linked to the operating microscope using 3 to 4 W of power in a pulsed mode. The arachnoid, like the dura mater, is opened in a crescentic fashion with the base of the flap toward the nondominant side of the spinal cord.

Next, the microlinked laser, defocused at 10 W of power with a pulse duration

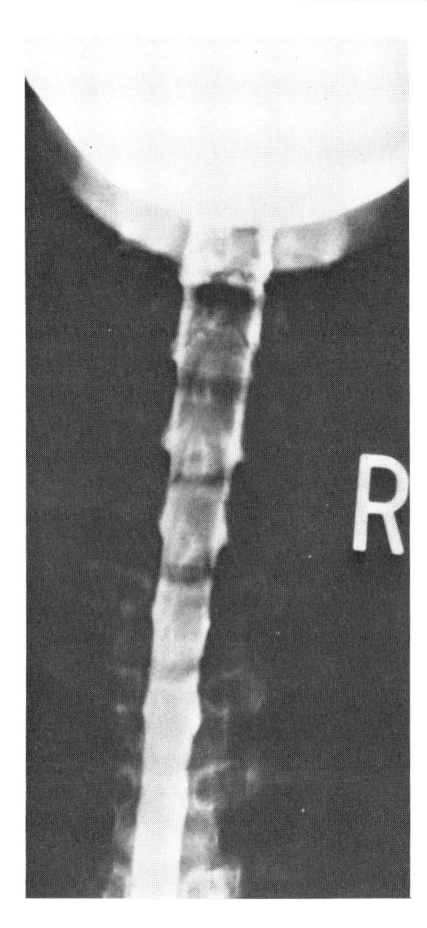

FIG 10-1.
Iophendylate injection (Pantopaque) myelography demonstrating diffuse widening of the cervicothoracic spinal cord consistent with a diagnosis of syringohydromyelia.

of 0.1 second and angled approximately 25 degrees from the vertical plane, is used to coagulate small vessels on the surface of the spinal cord at the dorsal root entry zone (DREZ). Thereafter, the laser is focused and, with 10 W of power still in a pulsed mode, the cord is fenestrated in the same area (Fig 10-7). Controlled respiratory arrest for up to 30 seconds at a time facilitates precise vaporization. As the fenestration progresses and the syrinx is entered, one sees spinal fluid egress from the syrinx cavity and the spinal cord collapse. Intraoperative SSEP monitoring often improves after the fenestration is made. Both an increase in amplitude and a decrease in latency of the evoked response is frequently seen. The entire fenestration is then enlarged with the laser to about 3 to 4 mm in diameter. No stints or shunts are placed in the opening. The arachnoid is closed in a separate layer with interrupted microsutures. An effort is made to keep the arachnoidal incision and suture line away from the fenestration. The dura mater and remainder of the wound are then closed in the usual fashion.

RESULTS

In the past 7 years, 21 patients have been treated for syringohydromyelia with CO_2 laser fenestration of the spinal cord (Table 10–1). Most patients were young adults, and male subjects outnumbered female subjects almost two to one. The duration of symptoms before surgery ranged from 1 month to 18 years, but over 40% of patients had symptoms for less than 1 year. Most of the cases of syringohydromyelia were of the communicating type. In two early patients, however, the type was never determined because the Pantopaque myelogram was not performed in both the prone and supine positions to document whether or not a Chiari I malformation was present. In our series, the syrinx typically occurred in the cervical and upper thoracic regions of the spinal cord. Scoliosis and fractures were the most commonly associated bony anomalies. Nine patients had no bony abnormality whatsoever. There were no instances of basilar impression or occipitalization of the atlas. Concomitant syringobulbia was suspected, though not documented radiographically, in three patients with nystagmus. Preoperative CT scans of the brain were normal in all patients.

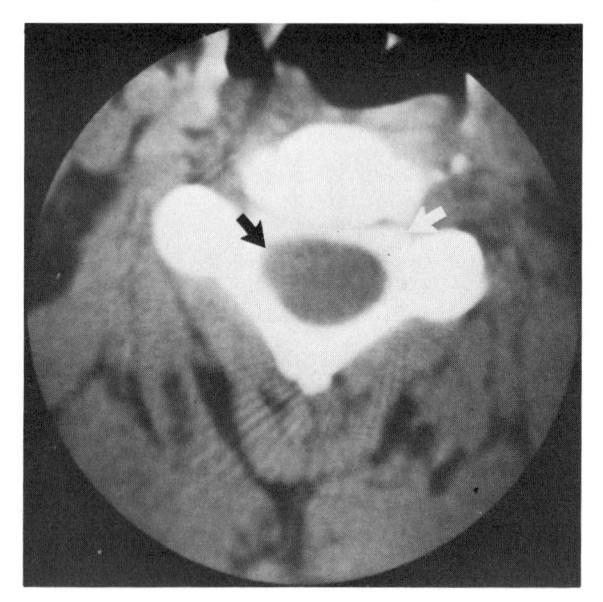

FIG 10–2.
Computed tomography of the cervical spine immediately following metrizamide myelography demonstrating an enlarged spinal cord (*black arrow*) surrounded by a column of metrizamide (*white arrow*).

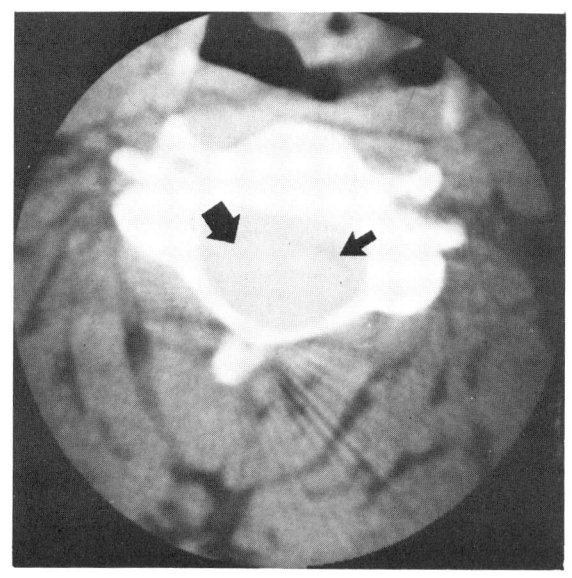

FIG 10-3.
Delayed computed tomography of the cervical spine following metrizamide myelography demonstrating influx of metrizamide into the syrinx cavity (*large arrow*) surrounded by a thin ribbon of cervical spinal cord (*small arrow*).

A good surgical result occurs in the treatment of syringohydromyelia if the patient's symptoms and signs improve postoperatively or if a progressive deterioration is halted. If the patient is not deteriorating and is unchanged postoperatively, a good surgical result cannot necessarily be claimed owing to the marked variability in the natural history of the disease process.

The vast majority of our patients initially improved, both subjectively and objectively, following surgery (see Table 10-1). One patient (patient 19) developed a severe wound infection and deteriorated neurologically. There have been nine recurrences, however, ranging from 6 to 54 months postoperatively, with an average time of recurrence of 29 months. Disease in a single patient (patient 4) recurred twice, at 16 and 32 months postoperatively. Three patients were refenestrated with the CO_2 laser at a different spinal level. Two of these patients have done well for 54 and 27 months, respectively. The third patient (patient 4) did well for 16 months, then had recurrence again and underwent syringoperitoneal shunting. Two patients received a syringoperitoneal shunt at the time of their recurrence, and another patient developed intercurrent hydrocephalus along with his recurrent syrinx and had a ventriculoperitoneal shunt placed. In three patients, interestingly, the spinal cord collapsed as CSF egressed from the subarachnoid space at the time of reoperation. This possibly indicates that the fenestration was still patent and that the CSF pathways were incompetent and incapable of keeping the syrinx decompressed. These three patients, therefore, received subarachnoid-peritoneal shunts.

There was no mortality in this series, and, aside from the one wound infection, surgical morbidity was minimal. It usually consisted of a frequently transient dermatomal hypesthesia corresponding to the site of laser fenestration at the DREZ.

CONCLUSIONS

Numerous surgical modalities have been employed over the years in the treatment of syringohydromyelia. There have been few extensive follow-up studies, however, and no single surgical procedure has been consistently shown to be the most effective over the long term. The goal of any procedure is to communicate the syrinx with functional CSF pathways. It was initially theorized that

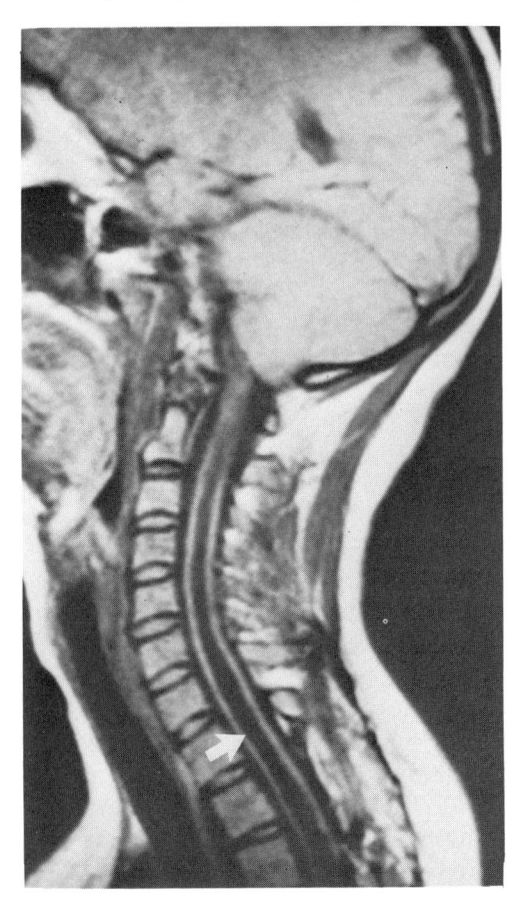

FIG 10–4.
Magnetic resonance imaging of the cervicothoracic spinal cord indicating a large syrinx cavity (*arrow*) within the cord.

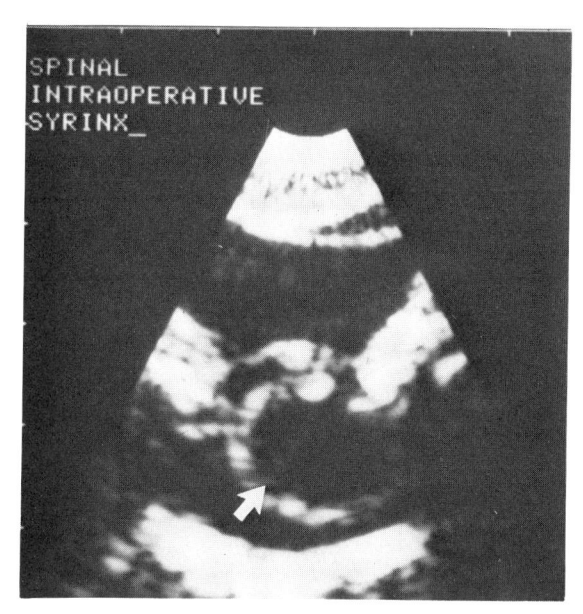

FIG 10-5.
Intraoperative ultrasonography (axial view) showing a large symmetrical syrinx cavity (*arrow*) within the spinal cord.

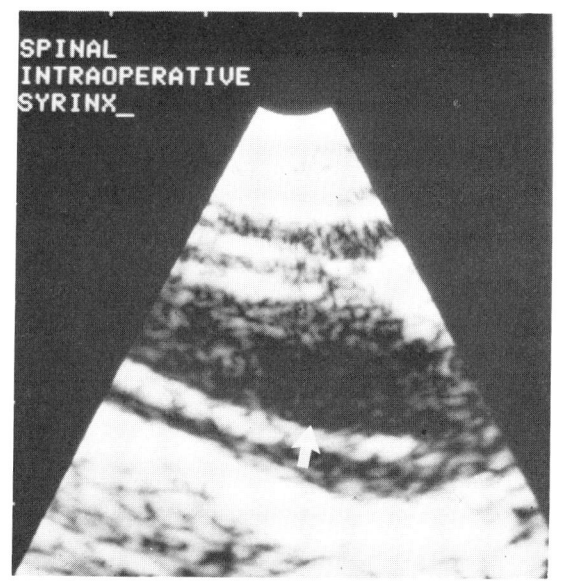

FIG 10-6.
Intraoperative ultrasonography (sagittal view) again showing a syrinx cavity (*arrow*) within the spinal cord.

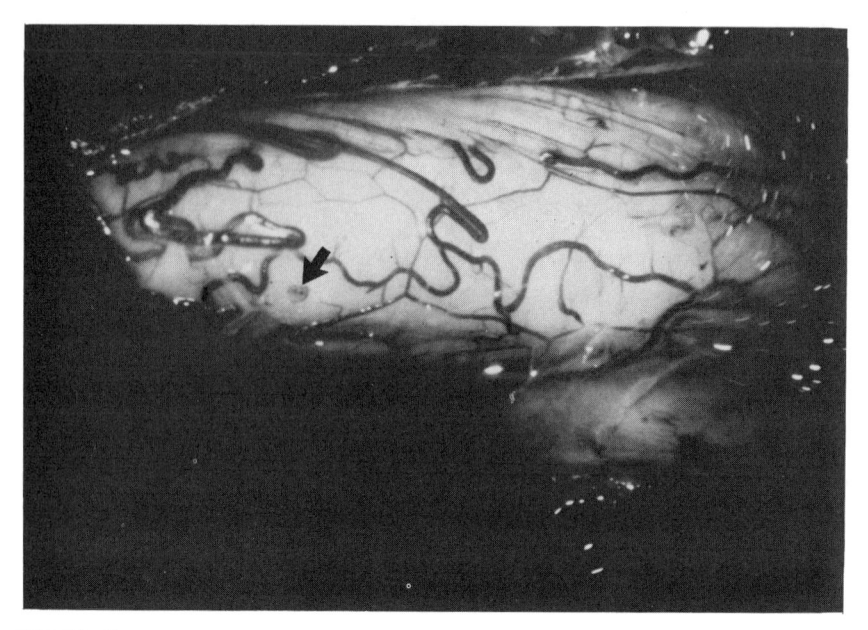

FIG 10–7.
Intraoperative view of an enlarged cervicothoracic spinal cord demonstrating early laser fenestration (*arrow*) of the syrinx cavity at the dorsal root entry zone.

laser syringostomy would be more safe and effective than other operative procedures heretofore attempted. The procedure is safe because it avoids spinal cord manipulation and the implantation of foreign bodies. It also affords uninterrupted intraoperative electrophysiologic monitoring of spinal cord function. The safety of the procedure is confirmed by the absence of mortality and very low morbidity. The effectiveness of the procedure was postulated to come from actually vaporizing and removing a small portion of the spinal cord rather than simply incising the tissue. It was hoped that this would reduce scarring and help maintain patency. On long-term follow-up, however, the effectiveness of laser syringostomy has not been proved, and syringohydromyelia remains an enigmatic, challenging, and often frustrating condition that confronts the neurosurgeon.

PAIN

The treatment of chronic intractable pain will occasionally call for neuroablative procedures. Because the duration of success of such operations is usually limited, they are primarily used for pain due to neoplasia rather than for deafferentation pain and other pain of neurogenic origin. Since these procedures are inherently destructive and carry a significant risk of disagreeable sensory phenomena as well as added neurologic deficit, they are customarily reserved for

TABLE 10–1.
Syringohydromyelia: Patient Data

PATIENT NO./AGE, YR/SEX	DURATION OF SYMPTOMS,	TYPE*	SITE	ASSOCIATED BONY ANOMALIES	SYRINGOBULBIA	DATE OF SURGERY	OUTCOME	FOLLOW-UP, MO
1/37/F	10.0	?	C-1-T-3	Scoliosis	–	12/79, 6/84	+then –	81
2/8/M	5.5	Com	C-1-T-3	Scoliosis	+	4/80	+	77
3/19/M	0.2	Noncom	C-1-L-2	Gunshot wound	–	10/80	+	71
4/45/F	12.0	?	C-1-T-8	...	–	1/81, 9/83, 1/85	+then –	68
5/30/F	0.2	Com	C-1-T-5	...	–	9/81, 3/82	+then –	60
6/44/F	0.4	Com	C-1-T-4	Multiple	–	1/82	+	56
7/39/F	0.3	Com	C-2-T-8	...	+	5/82, 5/86	+then –	52
8/9/M	0.6	Com	C-3-T-2	Spina bifida	–	5/82, 10/83	+then –	52
9/25/M	0.1	Noncom	C-7-T-2	Stab Wound	–	8/82	+	49
10/24/M	0.3	Noncom	C-2-T-2	Fracture	–	10/82	+	47
11/31/M	1.2	Com	C-4-T-6	Scoliosis	–	10/82, 2/85	+then –	47
12/42/M	7.0	Com	C-2-T-2	...	–	6/83	+	39
13/19/M	4.0	Noncom	C-2-T-5	...	–	9/83, 1/86	+then –	36
14/46/M	3.5	Com	C-2-L-1	Gunshot wound	–	2/84, 8/86	+then –	31
15/29/F	9.0	?	C-2-T-1	...	–	4/84	+	29
16/34/F	12.0	Com	C-1-T-9	...	–	11/84, 6/86	+then –	22
17/45/M	0.5	Com	T-4-T-10	Fracture	–	5/85	+	16
18/47/F	3.0	Noncom	C-3-T-1	Osteomyelitis	+	5/85	+	16
19/53/M	18.0	Noncom	C-6-T-6	...	–	5/85	–	16
20/35/M	2.0	Noncom	C-1-T-10	Fracture	–	11/85	+	10
21/25/M	0.7	Com	C-2-T-6	...	–	6/86	+	3

*Com indicates communicating; noncom, noncommunicating.

those patients who have failed all reasonable radiotherapeutic, pharmacologic, psychosocial, and neuroaugmentative attempts at pain control.

Lasers, thus far, have principally been used to modulate pain at the spinal-cord level. There has been modest clinical experience using CO_2 and argon lasers for anterolateral cordotomy, commissural myelotomy, and DREX lesions. Although there has been no proof that laser ablation of neural tissue affords any better pain relief than conventional techniques, some suggest, at least for DREZ lesions, that it provides relief with fewer complications.[18-20]

Somewhat limited personal experience using a CO_2 laser to affect pain at the spinal-cord level will be discussed in this section as well as some theoretical considerations including laser hypophysectomy, rhizotomy, and neurectomy. However, not enough cases have yet been accumulated to present a meaningful series.

ANTEROLATERAL CORDOTOMY

Although anterolateral cordotomy can be performed percutaneously,[21] occasionally an open approach is necessary or more desirable. In 1964, Cloward[22] provided a detailed description of cervical cordotomy by means of an anterior approach to the cervical spine. Hardy and associates,[23] in 1974, reaffirmed this approach, emphasizing use of the operating microscope to perform the procedure.

By linking the CO_2 laser to the operating microscope, an anterolateral cordotomy can be done in a quick and virtually bloodless fashion. With the laser defocused at 5 to 10 W of power using a pulse duration of 0.1 second, the pial surface is first coagulated. The cord is then vaporized to the desired depth with the laser in focus. The depth of the lesion can be assessed with microprobes. The dura is closed with microsuture using hemoclips. A bone dowel is taken from the analgesic hip. Although the procedure can be performed using simple diskectomy and a vertebral spreader, the dura in this instance is impossible to close and CSF fistulae are likely to result. As in all spinal cord procedures, SSEP monitoring is carried out continuously.

The laser has not been used for posterior approaches to the spinothalamic tract.

COMMISSURAL MYELOTOMY

Neoplastic pain of the lower extremities and pelvis can often be effectively treated by section of the anterior commissure at the caudal end of the spinal cord. Recent reviews by Cook and Kawakami[24] and by King[25] have not only demonstrated the potential effectiveness of the procedure but have also pointed out its limitations, especially long-term. Ascher[26] was the first to use the CO_2 laser for commissural myelotomy.

Our group prefers a four-level laminectomy, generally T-10 to L-1. After the dura and arachnoid are opened, the posterior median sulcus is identified under the operating microscope. It is best to open the sulcus with sharp microdissection, as using the laser at this point may distort the narrow cleavage plane. As the sulcus is opened, the central canal and anterior commissure are encountered. The posterior columns are held apart either with fine retractors or with pial retraction sutures. The laser is focused at approximately 5 W of power with a pulse duration of 0.1 second, and the anterior commissure is vaporized until the anterior median fissure is identified. Identification of the fissure is usually not difficult, especially its more rostral portion. Vaporization of the commissure is veritably bloodless.

Thus far, there has been no opportunity to perform this procedure at more rostral levels of the spinal cord.

DREZ LESIONS

Nashold and coworkers[27,28] first described DREZ lesions as treatment for intractable pain due primarily to cervical root avulsion and traumatic paraplegia. Using a radio frequency (RF) generator, they obtained impressive results for pain relief but encountered a significant amount of postoperative ipsilateral motor and proprioceptive impairment. In 1983, Levy et al.[18] suggested that the CO_2 laser might be superior to the RF generator for making such lesions. They believed the laser was faster and more precise and would result in fewer complications. Powers and coworkers,[20] in an experimental and clinical study using principally an argon laser, basically concurred. More recently, Levy et al.[19] described an experimental study in which laser DREZ lesions were found to be much more precise and less variable than RF lesions. In summary, the significant contribution of Nashold and associates to the treatment of certain types of deafferentation pain and other forms of neurogenic pain seems to have been advanced by laser technology.

The DREZ is often not readily identifiable in previously traumatized spinal cords. Its position can accurately be assessed, however, by observing normal rootlets both adjacent and contralateral to the involved area. After the operating microscope and laser are angled approximately 25 degrees from the vertical plane, the laser is slightly defocused and, at 10 W of power with a 0.1-second pulse duration, the DREZ is coagulated. The lesions are then made with the laser focused. About two to three bursts of energy are needed to produce a lesion 2 mm deep. The actual depth can be assessed with a fine tear-duct probe. The lesions are made 2 mm apart so that they coalesce to form a continuum of vaporization. Again, deliberate respiratory pauses of up to 30 seconds greatly facilitate optical focusing and precise lesioning.

HYPOPHYSECTOMY, RHIZOTOMY, AND NEURECTOMY

Tindall et al.[29,30] and others have shown hypophysectomy to be efficacious in both reduction of pain and actual objective remission of disseminated metastases from breast and prostate carcinoma. Significant pain relief can also be expected in some patients with widespread nonendocrine-sensitive tumors.[31] Although hypophysectomy can be performed by a variety of direct and stereotaxic methods, the direct transsphenoidal route still seems to be the one most widely used. Theoretically, in situ transsphenoidal laser vaporization of the pituitary gland and its stalk, if necessary, could offer some safety advantages over more standard techniques.

Ascher[32] and Saunders and coworkers[33] have suggested that laser neurectomy may reduce the chance of painful neuroma formation. In a recent article by Fischer et al.,[34] however, no significant differences in neuroma formation could be found histologically in rats after sciatic nerve section with a CO_2 laser vs. a scalpel. Although species differences could play a role, there are as yet no large long-term clinical studies to suggest that laser neurectomy is superior to other techniques. The same applies for rhizotomy.

SUMMARY

The physical properties and tissue interaction characteristics of the CO_2 laser make it, theoretically, an ideal instrument for neuroablation. The results of its use in our hands for the treatment of syringohydromyelia, however, have been disappointing, and this remains a frustrating condition to correct surgically. Only limited experience has been gained thus far in use of the laser for pain modulation at the spinal-cord level, but the initial results have been encouraging. Other potential uses of the laser for neuroablation have been mentioned. The concept is good; more experience, both laboratory and clinical, is needed.

REFERENCES
1. Brain WR: *Brain's Diseases of the Nervous System.* New York, Oxford University Press, 1977.
2. Greenfield JG: *Greenfield's Neuropathology.* Chicago, Year Book Medical Publishers, 1976.
3. Gardner WJ: Hydrodynamic mechanism of syringomyelia: Its relationship to myelocele. *J Neurol Neurosurg Psychiatry* 1965; 28:247–259.
4. Williams B: The distending force in the production of "communicating syringomyelia." *Lancet* 1969; 2:189–193.
5. Conway LW: Hydrodynamic studies in syringomyelia. *J Neurosurg* 1967; 27:501–514.
6. Williams B: Current concepts of syringomyelia. *Br J Hosp Med* 1970; 4:331–342.
7. Gardner WJ, Bell HS, Poolos PN, et al: Terminal ventriculostomy for syringomyelia. *J Neurosurg* 1977; 46:609–617.

8. Love JG, Olafson RA: Syringomyelia: A look at surgical therapy. *J Neurosurg* 1966; 24:714–718.
9. Tator CH, Meguro K, Rowed DW: Favorable results with syringosubarachnoid shunts for the treatment of syringomyelia. *J Neurosurg* 1982; 56:517–523.
10. Hankinson J: The surgical treatment of syringomyelia. *Adv Tech Stand Neurosurg* 1978; 5:127–151.
11. Barbaro NM, Wilson CB, Gutin PH, et al: Surgical treatment of syringomyelia: Favorable results with syringoperitoneal shunting. *J Neurosurg* 1984; 61:531–538.
12. Barnett HJM, Foster JB, Hudgson P: *Syringomyelia*. Philadelphia, WB Saunders Co, 1973.
13. Baker HL Jr: Myelographic examination of the posterior fossa with positive contrast medium. *Radiology* 1963; 81:791–801.
14. Forbes W St C, Isherwood I: Computed tomography in syringomyelia and the associated Arnold Chiari type I malformation. *Neuroradiology* 1978; 15:73–78.
15. Aubin ML, Vignaud J, Jardin C, et al: Computed tomography in 75 clinical cases of syringomyelia. *Am J Neuroradiol* 1981; 2:199–204.
16. Pojunas K, Williams AL, Daniels DL, et al: Syringomyelia and hydromyelia: Magnetic resonance evaluation. *Radiology* 1984; 153:679–683.
17. Lee BCP, Zimmerman RD, Manning JJ et al: MR imaging of syringomyelia and hydromyelia. *AJNR* 1985; 6:221–228.
18. Levy WJ, Nutkiewicz A, Ditmore QM, et al: Laser-induced dorsal root entry zone lesions for pain control: Report of three cases. *J Neurosurg* 1983; 59:884–886.
19. Levy WJ, Gallo C, Watts C: Comparison of laser and radiofrequency dorsal root entry zone lesions in cats. *Neurosurgery* 1985; 16:327–330.
20. Powers SK, Adams JE, Edwards MSB, et al: Pain relief from dorsal root entry zone lesions made with argon and carbon dioxide microsurgical lasers. *J Neurosurg* 1984; 61:841–847.
21. Mullan S, Harper PV, Hekmatpanah J, et al: Percutaneous interruption of spinal pain tract by means of a strontium needle. *J Neurosurg* 1963; 20:931–939.
22. Cloward RB: Cervical cordotomy by the anterior approach: Technique and advantages. *J Neurosurg* 1964; 21:19–25.
23. Hardy J, Leclercq TA, Mercky F: Microsurgical cordotomy by the anterior approach: Technical note. *J Neurosurg* 1974; 41:640–643.
24. Cook AW, Kawakami Y: Commissural myelotomy. *J Neurosurg* 1977; 47:1–6.
25. King RB: Anterior commissurotomy for intractable pain. *J Neurosurg* 1977; 47:7–11.
26. Ascher PW: Longitudinal medial myelotomy with the laser in *Proceedings of the Sixth International Congress of Neurological Surgery*. Sao Paulo, Brazil, 1977.
27. Nashold BS, Ostdahl RH: Dorsal root entry zone lesions for pain relief. *J Neurosurg* 1979; 51:59–69.
28. Nashold BS, Bullitt E: Dorsal root entry zone lesions to control central pain in paraplegics. *J Neurosurg* 1981; 55:414–419.
29. Tindall GT, Payne NS, Nixon DW: Transsphenoidal hypophysectomy for disseminated carcinoma of the prostate gland. *J Neurosurg* 1979; 50:275–282.
30. Schwarz M, Tindall GT, Nixon DW: Transsphenoidal hypophysectomy in disseminated breast cancer. *South Med J* 1981; 74:315–317.
31. Tindall GT, Nixon DW, Christy JH, et al: Pain relief in metastatic cancer other than breast and prostate gland following transsphenoidal hypophysectomy. *J Neurosurg* 1977; 47:659–662.

32. Ascher PW: Newest ultrastructural findings after the use of a CO_2 laser on CNS tissue. *Acta Neurochir Suppl* 1979; 28:572–581.
33. Saunders ML, Young HF, Becker DP, et al: The use of the laser in neurological surgery. *Surg Neurol* 1980; 14:1–10.
34. Fischer DW, Beggs JL, Shetter AG, et al: Comparative study of neuroma formation in the rat sciatic nerve after CO_2 laser and scalpel neurectomy. *Neurosurgery* 1983; 13:287–294.

11 Theoretical Neurosurgery

MATTHEW R. QUIGLEY, M. D.

JULIAN E. BAILES, M.D.

Less than a decade following the reintroduction of the carbon dioxide (CO_2) laser into clinical neurosurgery, the instrument has come into widespread use. Although this speaks for its usefulness and safety, a relative dearth of experimental work has preceded its utilization in the operating room. In addition, new laser sources such as the argon (Ar) and neodymium (Nd)-YAG are making their way into practice. Whereas the tissue response with the CO_2 laser is relatively uniform, depending on water content, the action of these other wavelengths is more a function of tissue pigmentation and blood flow so that their effects on tissue are not immediately obvious or easy to predict.

This chapter will deal with the basic laser-tissue interactions associated with the three laser sources utilized in neurosurgery: CO_2, Nd:YAG, and Ar. We shall rely primarily on controlled laboratory studies that illustrate the principles on which laser neurosurgery is founded. In addition, specific applications will be addressed, with relevant experimental and clinical studies cited.

EFFECT OF LASER SOURCES ON NEURAL TISSUES

BASIC MECHANISMS

Use of the laser in current clinical practice is almost totally restricted to the precise ablation of tissue by affording a delicate means of delivering controlled power into confined spaces. The action of the laser in these circumstances is effected by the conversion of light energy into heat energy at the point of impact. How this comes about is a function of the amount of light absorbed. Light not absorbed is scattered back toward the source and lost, or it penetrates deeper into the tissue. Theoretical calculations for tissue absorption of various wavelengths are based on experiments done with water, resting on the dubious assumption that this is the most important constituent of tissue. Absorption is expressed as a value termed the extinction length (L), which is the distance required to absorb 90% of incident light. These values are 0.3, 100, and 300 mm for CO_2, Nd:YAG, and Ar, respectively.[30] For the CO_2, this means that its interaction with tissue is based on its absorption by water, which occurs primarily on the surface with little scatter. For the Nd:YAG and Ar, the water analogy breaks down, for these wavelengths are avidly absorbed by pigments and blood.

Each organ will therefore have its own characteristic L value for different wavelengths. Wharen and associates[36] calculated an in vitro L in cat brain of 5.5 mm for Nd:YAG. In addition, whole blood had an absorption coefficient 100 times greater than did brain. They postulated that the in vivo L for brain should be even less than 5.5 mm owing to the effect of the circulating blood. This work also supports use of the Nd:YAG laser as a selectively coagulating instrument. Similar experiments comparing laser absorption in blood found relative penetration depths of 1:4.2 for Ar and Nd:YAG, respectively, indicating that Ar has an even greater affinity than Nd:YAG for hemoglobin pigments.[32] Boggan et al.[5] produced CO_2 and Ar brain lesions in rats at equal power densities and found similar depths of penetration (0.75 mm), with more edema associated with the CO_2 lasers as indicated by Evans blue staining. From these data they concluded that the in vivo absorption characteristics of the two wavelengths are probably similar.

In summary, the response of tissue to CO_2 laser light is an almost complete conversion of the laser energy into heat energy on the tissue surface, independent of pigmentation or blood content. The Nd:YAG and Ar lasers, however, will penetrate and scatter to various degrees based on specific tissue characteristics. In brain cortex, the action of the Ar is probably similar to that of the CO_2, whereas the Nd:YAG undoubtedly scatters and penetrates to a greater degree than the other two sources.

LESION SIZE

Intuitively, a laser lesion diameter should correspond to the laser spot size used and the depth to the power applied. Owing to the light scatter associated with different lasers, however, lesion characteristics will vary. The CO_2 laser lesion most closely approximates beam parameters. Boggan and associates[5] found that a CO_2 with a spot size of 0.45 mm produced a lesion 0.86 mm in diameter, contrasted to Ar producing a 0.65 mm defect with a 0.15 mm spot. Thus, relative to spot size, the Ar affected five times the amount of tissue the CO_2 laser affected. For the Nd:YAG, these discrepancies are even more pronounced. Beck et al.[3] reported a 2.4 mm beam creating a lesion with a 6.8 mm diameter. The geometry of the defect, they concluded, was energy dependent, the lesion depth being a function of the log of the energy (in watts or joules). This resulted in progressively wider lesions with increasing energies. Eggert et al.[10] confirmed the logarithmic relation between energy and depth of lesion and demonstrated that total lesion size varied with the log of energy applied. With the Nd:YAG laser, therefore, increased energy levels yield progressively less tissue ablation. The CO_2 lesion, on the other hand, does not widen with added energy but rather creates a fissure, the depth of which is related not to the power or energy, but rather the log of time applied to the tissue.[3]

TEMPERATURE CHANGES

Few reports in the literature document the thermal effects of lasers in vivo.

Wharen et al.[36] measured the temperature in cat brains 5 and 10 mm below an Nd:YAG lesion. Although relatively large temperature swings occurred at 5 mm (30°C for 20 W, 8 seconds) the effects were negligible at 1 cm. Burke and associates[8] studied this more precisely using a stereotaxic device to position their probe and found tremendous temperature increases with even brief exposure of Nd:YAG. Within 1 mm of an Nd:YAG lesion of 25 W for 0.5 seconds with 0.4 mm spot, the temperatures exceeded boiling. They compared this with the CO_2 laser and found only minimal (3°C) thermal changes. The thermal spread due to scatter, therefore, is very significant when carefully sought.

HISTOLOGIC CHANGES

As all laser lesions are thermally induced, the basic histologic morphology for all wavelengths is the same.[9] The stereotyped lesion, if energy levels are high enough, consists of an area of vaporization (or steam formation) surrounded by carbonization. Adjacent to this is a zone of coagulation necrosis, which may manifest gross honeycombing close to the lesion center, becoming more homogenous at the periphery. This is surrounded by a zone of edema. The area of coagulation necrosis is greatest for lasers with the most scatter, extending up to 1 mm for Nd:YAG and Ar. This zone is thought important for hemostasis as it contains many coagulated small vessels.

Following acute injury, the lesion increases in size, primarily by enlargement of the coagulation necrosis and edematous zone, peaking at 16 hours.[10,37] In subsequent days, the area of necrosis becomes the site for the accumulation of macrophage and capillary proliferation. The edema subsides by 3 days, and eventually the chronic lesion shows only a thin rim of cicatrices filled with lipid-laden macrophages.[9]

The microvasculature surrounding these lesions has been studied extensively. Boggan et al.[5] investigated Evans blue staining following CO_2 and Ar lesions and found that a half hour following injury, staining about the CO_2 lesion was five times that about the Ar. By 24 hours, both lesions had only faint staining. Toya and coworkers[35] studied the epicerebral microcirculation with fluorescein angiography. Using high-speed photography, they observed a 1.0 to 1.5-mm nonfilling strip immediately following CO_2 laser lesioning. Adjacent to this was another 1.0 to 1.5-mm area where fluorescein extravasation was noted, and circulation time was delayed as well. The circulation was normal 2 to 3 mm distal to the lesion.

Other investigators have also noted subtle changes in the periphery of laser lesions. Burke and associates[7] found loss of functioning catecholamine fibers surrounding the coagulation necrosis zone following Nd:YAG irradiation. This extended the destruction of physiologically intact tissue by a factor of 0.3 beyond that which appeared viable on routine hematoxylin-eosin staining. In contrast,

CO_2 lesions demonstrated functioning terminals abutting the coagulum. By three days, the Nd:YAG matched the CO_2. As more subtle criteria are used, the histologic, vascular, and physiochemical alterations associated with various wavelengths are seen to extend beyond the putative boundaries of the lesion.

PHYSIOLOGIC EFFECTS

A few investigators have addressed the systemic effects of lesioning the brain with laser. Tiznado et al.[33,34] found an almost linear relation between laser power and raised intracranial pressure 24 hours following injury when all other factors were controlled. Interestingly, this could be blocked with the administration of steroids, an effect associated with decreased cortical water content. Work in our laboratories[6] has addressed the effect of cranial laser irradiation on the renin-angiotensin system. We found a significant decline in lung and serum levels of angiotensin converting enzyme and a significant rise in lung plasminogen activator 24 hours following a brief Nd:YAG exposure (35 W, 0.1 second, 1.5 mm spot) to rat cortex. Similar CO_2 lesioning produced no changes compared with controls.

It is clear that the investigations of the systemic and distant effects of laser exposure to brain are only in their infancy. We can no longer assume that this is an isolated thermal interaction, especially as perturbations in a wide range of systems are discovered.

SPECIFIC APPLICATIONS

DORSAL ROOT ENTRY ZONE LESIONS

Following the lead of Nashold et al.,[21,23] who produced dorsal root entry zone (DREZ) lesions by radiofrequency (RF) techniques for the relief of intractable pain, Levy et al.[17] were the first to report using the CO_2 laser to achieve spinal DREZ lesions. They cited shorter operating time and precise lesioning as the advantages of this alternative method, as the RF procedure had been implicated in a significant incidence of contralateral motor weakness. Powers and coworkers[24] applied the laser to make cat DREZ lesions and found minimal somatosensory evoked potential changes with two cats developing unilateral but transient monopareses. The histologic findings of the lesions were as previously described for brain cortex, and none involved the corticospinal tract. These investigators also reported their clinical series of 21 patients with a variety of pain syndromes. Clinical response, as defined by 50% or greater pain relief, was achieved in 17 of 21 patients initially but dropped to 14 of 21 on follow-up. No patient experienced any motor impairment. They deemed these results comparable to RF lesioning, with a lower complication rate. In a subsequent study, Levy and associates[18] compared both laser and RF lesions in the cat spinal cord. They found that when adopting standard clinical procedures, the RF lesion was twice as large and, on repeated applications, had 3 times the variability of the CO_2 laser applications. Whether both these lesions would have produced comparable pain relief is a matter of conjecture. The only drawbacks to the laser technique were technical shortcomings: alignment of the helium-neon aiming beam and laser-microscope focus discrepancies.

NEURECTOMY

Some investigators[1,30] have suggested that the laser is a superior tool for performing neurectomy, as the laser "seals" the end of the nerve and prevents neuroma formation. Fischer et al.,[12] working with rat sciatic nerves, could find no advantage in CO_2 laser neurectomy vs. scalpel neurectomy. Histologically, they found the laser nerves had greater axonal densities and more giant cells compared with the conventionally done side. Thus, laser neurectomy in this model offered no advantages over present techniques.

ANEURYSM OBLITERATION

In a singular study, Maira et al.[19] reported the use of an Ar laser to treat experimentally produced aneurysms. Using both arterial and venous models, they tried a number of different techniques to effect obliteration. These included total aneurysmal photocoagulation, partial coagulation (one side only), and focal neck coagulation. The results were encouraging, with over half of the totally or partially exposed aneurysms being excluded from the circulation. Of interest was that seven of nine complete occlusions occurred weeks to months following irradiation and were due to the proliferative response of the aneurysm wall.

Fasano and associates[11] applied this to the clinical situation. They used the Nd:YAG laser to shrink an anterior communicating artery (ACA) aneurysm before clipping, and the Ar to shrink small ACA and internal carotid artery (ICA) aneurysms. Only the ACA aneurysm was smaller on repeated angiography, the ICA one being unchanged.

TISSUE WELDING

VESSELS

The first report of low-power laser energy being used to "weld" tissues together as opposed to vaporizing them was in a rat arterial anastomosis experimental model utilizing the Nd:YAG laser.[16] Because of the difficulty of the technique and large spot sizes of the Nd:YAG units,[25] other investigators constructed a low-power CO_2 unit with a 150-μm spot size and successfully anastomosed rat femoral arteries using three stay sutures and 70 to 80 mW of power applied in short bursts.[31] Subsequent articles from our laboratory have outlined the vessel histology associated with the laser technique[26,27] being a coagulation necrosis that heals by the accumulation of myofibroblasts and loss of the elastic laminae associated with significant intimal proliferation. The bursting strength of the laser anastomoses was found to be significantly lower than suture controls when examined 1 day to 1 week following the procedure. By 2 weeks, the groups were comparable.[28] A significant difficulty with the laser-assisted technique lies in the formation of aneurysms, which occurred almost 30% of the time in rat femoral arteries followed up for at least 1 week.[29] This may not be a problem in large vessels of a different species where the muscularis is thicker.[14,20]

NERVES

The experimental work dealing with CO_2 laser nerve welding is not as extensive as that concerned with vessels. Fischer et al.[13] performed 31 laser-assisted nerve anastomoses in the rat sciatic nerve and reexplored these 60 days later. They found a 13% nerve dehiscence rate among this group (vs. 0% for suture controls), but nerve action potentials were comparable to those in the suture cohort. In a follow-up morphometric study,[4] this same group demonstrated similar axon counts and fiber diameters distal to both suture and laser techniques. This model, however, employed laser power settings of 5 W with a 600-μm spot aimed tangential to the nerve. Using a CO_2 milliwatt laser set at 90 mW with a 150-μm spot, our group has shown significantly less neuroma formation with the laser vs. suture anastomosed nerves. Our dehiscence rate was comparable to that in the above study. Using end-to-end and interposition grafting techniques, we also showed similar nerve conduction velocities between laser and suture cohorts.[2]

DURA

As the situation often arises where a watertight dural closure in a confined space is required, the application of laser tissue welding techniques in this area seemed appropriate. We operated on a series of dogs, closing the spinal dura with either 4-0 nylon or the milliwatt laser, set at 100 mW with a 150-μm spot. The laser effected a watertight seal initially, but with a closure strength significantly less than that of suture. At 3 and 6 weeks, the healing process between the groups appeared similar histologically, but tensile strength could not be assessed.[15]

REFERENCES
1. Ascher PW: Newest ultrastructural findings after the use of a CO_2 laser on CNS tissue. *Acta Neurochir Suppl* 1979; 28:572–581.
2. Bailes JE, Quigley MR, Cerullo LJ, et al: Nerve anastomosis with lowpower CO_2 laser. *Proc Am Int Phys,* in press.
3. Beck OJ, Welske J, Schonberger JL, et al: Tissue changes following application of laser to the rabbit brain. *Neurosurg Rev* 1979;1:31–36.

4. Beggs JL, Fischer DW, Shetter AG: Comparative study of rat sciatic microepineurial anastomoses made with carbon dixoide laser and suture techniques: II. *Neurosurgery* 1986;18:266–269.
5. Boggan JE, Edwards MSB, Davis RL, et al: Comparison of the brain tissue response in rats to injury by argon and carbon dioxide lasers. *Neurosurgery* 1982; 11:609–616.
6. Brizio-Molteni L, Quigley M, Cerullo L, et al: Brain surface exposure to CO_2 and Nd:YAG laser application: Effect on pulmonary endothelium response in the rat. *Burn*, in press..
7. Burke LP, Rovin RA, Cerullo LJ, et al: Nd:YAG laser in neurosurgery; Jaffe (ed): in *Nd:YAG Laser in Medicine and Surgery*. New York; Elsevier North-Holland, Inc, 1983; pp 141–148.
8. Burke L, Rovin RA, Cerullo LJ, et al: Thermal effects of the Nd:YAG and carbon dioxide lasers on the central nervous system. *Lasers Surg Med* 1985; 5:67–71.
9. Edwards MSB, Boggan JE, Fuller TA: The laser in neurologic surgery. *J Neurosurg* 1983; 59:555–566.
10. Eggert HR, Kiessling M, Kleihues P: Time course and spatial distribution of Nd:YAG laser-induced lesions in the rat brain. *Neurosurgery* 1985; 16:443–448.
11. Fasano VA, Urciuoli R, Ponzio RM: Photocoagulation of cerebral arteriovenous malformations and arterial aneurysms with the Nd:YAG or argon laser: Preliminary results in 12 patients. *Neurosurgery* 1982; 11:754–760.
12. Fischer DW, Beggs JL, Shetter AG, et al: Comparative study of neuroma formation in rat sciatic nerve after CO_2 laser and scapel neurectomy. *Neurosurgery* 1983; 13:287–294.
13. Fischer DW, Beggs JL, Kenshalo DL, et al: Comparative study of microepineurial anastomoses with the use of CO_2 laser and suture techniques in rat sciatic nerves: I. *Neurosurgery* 1985; 17:300–308.
14. Frazier OH, Painvin GA, Morris JR: Laser-assisted microvascular anastomosis: Angiographic and anatopathologic studies on growing microvascular anastomoses: Preliminary report. *Surgery* 1985; 97:585–589.
15. Heiferman KS, Quigley MR, Cerullo LJ, et al: Dural welding with CO_2 laser, abstracted. *Lasers Surg Med* 1986; 6:207.
16. Jain KK: Sutureless microvascular anastomosis using a Nd:YAG laser. *J Microsurg* 1980; 1:436–439.
17. Levy WJ, Natkiewicz A, Ditmore QM, et al: Laser induced dorsal root entry zone lesions for pain control. *J Neurosurg* 1983; 59:884–886.
18. Levy WJ, Gallo C, Watts C: Comparison of laser and radiofrequency dorsal root entry zone lesions in cats. *Neurosurgery* 1985; 16:327–330.
19. Maira G, Mahr G, Panissett A, et al: Laser photocoagulation for treatment of experimental aneurysms. *J Microsurg* 1979; 1:137–147.
20. McCarthy WJ, Hartz RS, Yao JST, et al:; Vascular anastomosis with laser energy. *J Vasc Surg* 1986; 3:32–41.
21. Nashold BS, Urban B, Zorub DS: Phantom pain relief by focal destruction of the substantia gelatinosa of Rolando. *Adv Pain Res Ther* 1976; 1:959–963.
22. Nashold BS, Ostdahl RH: Dorsal root entry zone lesions for pain relief. *J Neurosurg* 1979; 51:59–69.
23. Nashold BS, Bullet E: Dorsal root entry zone lesions to control central pain in paraplegics. *J Neurosurg* 1981; 55:414–419.
24. Powers SK, Adams JE, Edwards MSB, et al: Pain relief from dorsal root entry zone

lesions made with argon and carbon dioxide microsurgical lasers. *J Neurosurg* 1984; 61:841–847.
25. Quigley MR, Bailes JE, Kwaan HC, et al: Laser-assisted vascular anastomosis. *Lancet* 1985; 1:334.
26. Quigley MR, Bailes JE, Kwaan HC, et al: Microvascular anastomosis using the milliwatt CO_2 laser. *Lasers Surg Med* 1985; 5:357–365.
27. Quigley MR, Bailes JE, Kwaan HC, et al: Histological comparison of suture versus laser-assisted vascular anastomosis. *Surg Forum* 1985; 36:500–510.
28. Quigley MR, Bailes JE, Kwaan HC, et al: Comparison of bursting strength between suture and laser anastomosed vessels. *Microsurgery* 1985; 6:229–232.
29. Quigley MR, Bailes JE, Kwaan HC, et al: Aneurysm formation following low power CO_2 laser assisted vascular anastomosis. *Neurosurgery* 1986; 18:292–299.
30. Saunders ML, Young HF, Becker DP, et al: The use of laser in neurologic surgery. *Surg Neurol* 1980; 14:1–10.
31. Serure A, Withers EH, Thomsen S, et al: Comparison of carbon dioxide laser-assisted microvascular anastomosis and conventional microvascular sutured anastomosis. *Surg Forum* 1983; 34:634–636.
32. Stokes LF, Auth DL, Tanaka D, et al: Biomedical utility of 1.34 μM Nd:YAG laser radiation. *IEEE Trans Biomed Eng* 1981; 28:297–299.
33. Tiznado E, James HE, Kemper C: Experimental carbon dioxide laser brain lesions and intracranial dynamics: I. *Neurosurgery* 1985; 16:5–8.
34. Tiznado EG, James HE, Moore S: Experimental carbon dioxide laser brain lesions and intracranial dynamics: II. *Neurosurgery* 1985; 16:454–457.
35. Toya S, Kawase T, Irsaka Y, et al: Acute effect of the carbon dioxide laser on the epicerebral microcirculation. *J Neurosurg* 1980; 53:193–197.
36. Wharen RE, Anderson RE, Scheithauer B, et al: The Nd:YAG laser in neurosurgery: I. Laboratory investigations: Dose related biological response of neural tissue. *J Neurosurg* 1984; 60:531–539.
37. Yamagami T, Handa H, Taheuchi J, et al: Histologic study of normal rat brain tissue after Nd:YAG laser irradiation. *Surg Neurol* 1985; 23:475–482.

12 Photochemotherapy

STEPHEN K. POWERS, M.D.

Current techniques of treating locally invasive malignant tumors such as gliomas include surgery, radiation therapy, chemotherapy, and immunotherapy. None of these, except perhaps the last modality, offers the possibility of selective destruction of tumor without injury to normal tissue. Photochemotherapy (PCT), also termed photodynamic therapy, is a relatively new technique for treating malignant tumors that depends on the light activation of a photoreactive drug, called a photosensitizer, that is selectively taken up or retained by the neoplasm. Assuming that the photosensitizer preferentially bonds to all tumor cells, PCT not only offers the possibility of selective killing of rapidly proliferating cells but is potentially effective against tumor cells in any phase of the cell cycle. Several criteria regarding the photosensitizer must be met for PCT to be effective: (1) selectivity for tumor tissue; (2) absence of systemic toxic reaction at doses required for photosensitization; (3) capacity to absorb wavelengths of light that are readily transmitted through the tissue being treated; and (4) ability to destroy malignant tissue efficiently when photoactivated.

In 1900, Raab[1] reported on the lethal effect of acridine orange dye on paramecium exposed to light. In 1903, the topical use of eosin and the white light for photosensitization of skin tumors was described by Tappenier and Jesionek and was the first report on the use of photosensitization for the treatment of cancer.[2] Since that time a wide range of photosensitizing drugs have been studied in vitro and in vivo to determine their usefulness for PCT of a variety of neoplasms.[2-10]

The effectiveness of a photosensitizer will depend on the degree of localization of the drug in the tumor, which in turn is related to its solubility and partition and transport characteristics, and to the biochemical and biophysical properties of the normal and tumor tissues. Also, the effectiveness of the photosensitizer will depend on the photophysical parameters of the sensitizer, which include the quantum yield, on the lifetimes and energies of the excited singlet and triplet states of the photosensitizer, as well as consideration of tumor geometry in assessing light delivery.

Although a number of photosensitizers have been considered for localization and phototherapy of tumors, the porphyrins have received the most attention. Fluorescence in implanted tumors in rats after the systemic injection of hematoporphyrin was first witnessed by Auler and Banzer in 1942.[11] In addition to neoplastic tissues, embryonic, lymphatic, and traumatized tissues were also shown to have binding affinity for porphyrins and metalloporphyrins.[12] In 1960, Lipson et al.[13] introduced hematoporphyrin derivative (HPD), a mixture of porphyrins prepared by acetylating hematoporphyrin with an acetic acid - sulfuric acid mixture followed by hydrolysis under basic or near-neutral conditions, as a better fluorescent tumor marker than hematoporphyrin. Excellent correlation between fluorescing sites at endoscopy and biopsy-proved malignant neoplasia was demonstrated with HPD.[14-17] A preliminary report by Diamond et al.[18] on the use of hematoporphyrin for PCT of malignant gliomas in rats appeared in 1972. Since that time, PCT with HPD has been used both experimentally[19-33] and clinically[34-52] in managing various benign and malignant superficially placed tumors. Carcinoma of the lung, transitional cell carcinoma of the bladder, and tumors involving the skin have been the major lesions treated with PCT. Though the response rates for treatment have been high, PCT using HPD has not been curative. More recently, clinical trials have begun to study the efficacy of PCT using HPD in treating malignant gliomas.[53-57] Preliminary results from these studies have demonstrated the relative safety of performing PCT in this rather desperate group of patients; however, patient outcome has not been improved. The following presentation is a summary of the current knowledge of the biochemical and biophysical basis of PCT, the current status of PCT in the treatment of brain tumors, and considerations for future improvements in PCT.

PHOTOSENSITIZER

Several chemical compounds are capable of photosensitizing malignant brain tumor cells. Those that have been studied include hematoporphyrin,[18] HPD,[53-66] rhodamine 123,[67,68] acridine orange,[69] pyrylium derivatives,[70] and phthalocyanines.[71-73] From among this group, HPD has been the most widely studied photosensitizer to date.

Hematoporphyrin derivative is a mixture of porphyrins (tetrapyrrolic pigments) that is formed by the acetic acid–sulfuric acid treatment of hematoporphyrin. The resultant porphyrin mixture, commercially known as Photofrin I (HPD$_1$), contains hematoporphyrin and dihematoporphyrin ether (DHE)[74]; DHE appears to be the principle component of HPD responsible for in vivo photosensitization (Fig 12–1).[75] However, Moan et al.[76] conclude that the least polar components of HPD analyzed by high-performance liquid chromatography are the major components for photosensitization (Fig 12–2). The nonpolar components would exist as large aggregate molecules in aqueous solutions with a molecular weight of over 12,000 daltons. Using gel filtration, DHE has been isolated from HPD$_1$ to produce a commercially available material known as Photofrin II (HPD$_2$), which contains 90% DHE. Because of the instability of DHE in solution there is serious question regarding the actual purity of DHE in HPD$_2$.

Hematoporphyrin derivative can sensitize the photo-oxidation of many kinds of biologically important molecules. Since the photoactivation spectrum usually corresponds to the absorption spectrum of the photosensitizer, HPD can be activated by most visible light owing to its broad range of light absorption. When

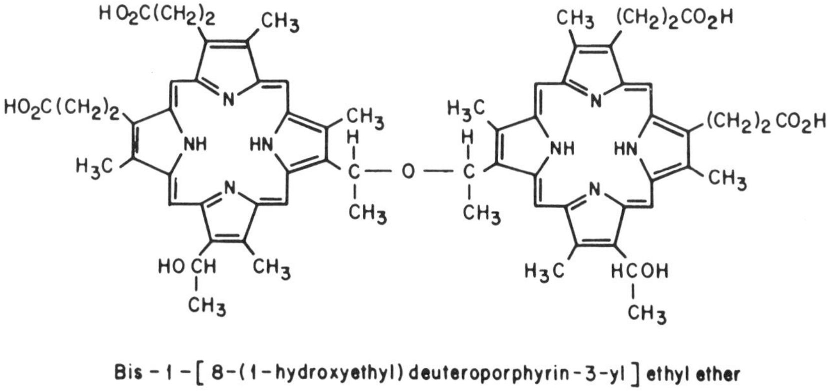

Bis-1-[8-(1-hydroxyethyl)deuteroporphyrin-3-yl] ethyl ether

FIG 12-1.
Chemical structure of dihematoporphyrin ether.

illuminated, HPD will absorb light energy and be transformed to an excited singlet state. Red fluorescence is seen with radiative decay from the excited singlet state. Transformation of the excited singlet-state HPD to the excited triplet state can occur by so-called intersystem crossover. Triplet-state lifetimes range over several hundred microseconds. During this time, triplet-state porphyrins can transfer energy to ground-state oxygen (which is in the triplet state) to produce excited singlet-state oxygen, which is chemically reactive. This is called a type II photo-oxidation process. A type I photo-oxidative process may occur instead if the triplet-state porphyrin transfers an electron to a molecule of oxygen to yield a superoxide (O_2^-) radical. In addition, the triplet-state porphyrin may react directly with certain biomolecules to initiate other free-radical processes. The ability to generate excited singlet oxygen is directly related to the length of porphyrin's triplet lifetime.[77]

It is unclear at present how HPD and the other porphyrins enter mammalian cells. It is assumed that HPD diffuses into cells, although it is recognized that active and passive transport processes as well as pinocytosis and phagocytosis may be involved. Porphyrin migration within cells as a function of incubation time has been demonstrated by the variable sites of intracellular damage following photoradiation for different periods between incubation and illumination.[78] The relative affinity of the various porphyrins for subcellular structures depends on their lipid solubility.[79]

In vitro studies show that the plasma membrane is the main site of porphyrin-sensitized photodamage.[80-86] Photoinduced alterations in the cell membrane include inactivation of membrane enzymes, cross-linking of membrane proteins, alterations in membrane permeability, damage to transport systems, and cell lysis. With longer incubation times, porphyrins will localize to the mitochondria, microsomes, and lysosomes and sensitize photodamage in those areas.[87-90] Occasionally structural changes are produced.[91] Oxygen-dependent and hypoxic cells are extremely resistant to the lethal effects of HPD and light.[92,93] This suggests that hypoxic areas in tumors may limit HPD phototherapy.

Why HPD preferentially localizes to tumors is still largely unknown. Evidence supports the concept that differences in the extracellular environment between neoplastic and normal tissue, such as vascular permeability, lack of adequate lymphatic drainage, and nonspecific binding of proteins to stromal elements, are responsible for the selective uptake or retention of HPD and other porphyrins within tumor.[84-89] Hematoporphyrin derivative accumulation in the stroma and

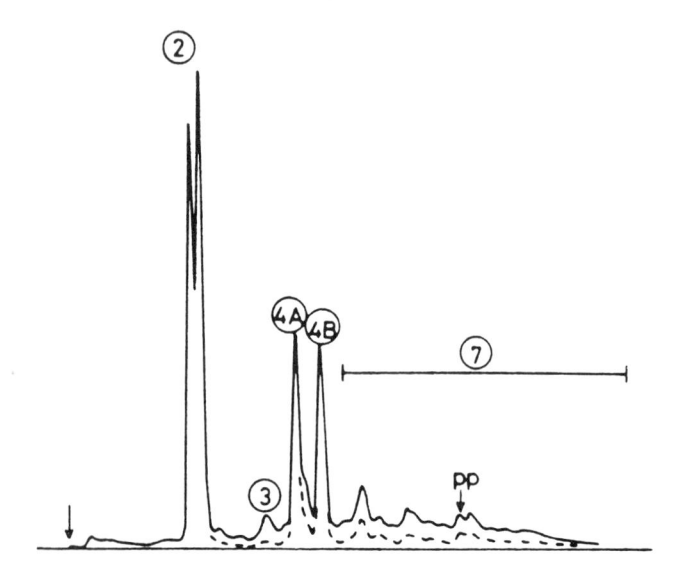

FIG 12-2.
High-performance liquid chromatogram of hematoporphyrin derivative (HPD); optical absorption was recorded at 393 nm. The relative amounts of different components present in HPD and in hematoporphyrin (HP) treated for 1 hour with 0.1N sodium hydroxide, and the relative sensitizing efficiency of the two porphyrin mixtures, are as follows (From Moan J, Christensen T, Jacobson PB: Porphyrin-sensitized photoinactivation of cells in vitro, in Dorion DR, Gomer CJ (eds): *Porphyrin Localization and Treatment of Tumors.* New York, Alan R Liss, 1984, pp 419-442. Reproduced by permission).

	RELATIVE AMOUNT OF COMPONENT			RELATIVE SENSITIZING EFFICIENCY
	2	4A + 4B	7	
HP	2.1	0.5	0.38	0.35
HPD	0.9	0.6	1.0	1.0

in macrophages of tumors has been shown autoradiographically.[94] Using tritiated HPD, Little et al.[60] found twice the concentration of HPD_1 in intracerebrally implanted 9L gliosarcomas compared with normal brain in the rat at 24 hours after intravenous injection (10 mg/kg) and 20 times the concentration of HPD_2 in the tumor compared with normal brain at 24 hours after intravenous injection (7.5 mg/kg). For identical intravenous dosages of HPD_1 and HPD_2 (7.5 mg/kg), the concentration of HPD_2 in tumor was 1.5 times greater than of HPD_1 at 24 hours after injection. Wharen et al.[61] compared levels of HPD in normal tissues and ethylnitrosourea-induced experimental brain tumors in rats using fluorescence and radioactive labeling assays. Very little HPD was present in normal brain at 24 hours after injection (0.1 μg/g) in contrast to higher levels in the experimental tumors (0.3 to 10.9 μg/g). The HPD concentration was also determined by fluorescent assay in three human gliomas from patients who were given 5 mg/kg of HPD intravenously at 24 to 48 hours before. The values at 24 hours were 1.7 and 2.5 μg/mL, whereas the concentration fell to 0.1 μg/mL at 48 hours. These quantitative studies suggest a therapeutic ratio of approximately 20:1 based on the concentration of HPD in tumor vs. brain at 24 hours.

Analysis of the distribution of HPD in rat 9L gliosarcoma brain tumors by digital video fluorescent microscopy at 24 hours after injection of the drug intravenously shows that only 33% to 44% of the tumor is fluorescent.[59] The patchy pattern of fluorescence that was seen with areas of intense fluorescent staining around blood vessels and sinusoidal vascular channels suggests that HPD is distributed in a perivascular pattern. Maximum fluorescence in normal brain was seen in blood vessels at the pia - gray matter margin at 4 hours after injection.[59] Vascular injury evidenced by vessel engorgement, thrombosis, and extravasation of red cells was noted throughout the tumors after exposure to light.

Because of its large size and protein binding, HPD does not cross the blood-brain barrier (BBB).[95,96] It diffuses into tumor areas where the BBB may be altered and areas of the brain that are devoid of the BBB, such as the pituitary, area postrema, pineal gland, choroid plexus, and meninges.[61-64] Hematoporphyrin derivative thus leaks out into the intercellular space in areas of capillary permeability and is taken up or retained by both tumor and normal cells in the area. Tumor cells that are removed by distance from the BBB defect would not be expected to incorporate HPD and thus would not be photosensitive. In addition, the unselective staining of normal brain tissue by HPD in the region of BBB defect adjacent to the tumor mass could lead to injury of these cells during photoillumination. Photochemotherapy with HPD does not affect tumor cell clonogenicity even at doses that produce macroscopic tumor destruction.[97] It is currently believed that tumor destruction by HPD and light is not cell specific and instead results from damage to the tumor circulation and treatment-induced changes in tumor physiology.[59,65,94,97] Further concern with the use of HPD has arisen from reports that the nonfluorescing, intact, nontumor-bearing brain tissue from HPD-treated mice and rats may be injured following nonthermal levels of light exposure.[58-98]

Investigators are currently studying other agents for their potential role as photosensitizers in the treatment of malignant gliomas and other tumors. Rhodamine 123 is a vital dye that has been widely used in the study of living mitochondria by cell biologists.[99] It accumulates in the mitochondria of tumor cells owing to prolonged retention that is the result of its cationic charge and the increased intramitochondrial negativity of the transformed cell.[100-103] Normal brain does not accumulate rhodamine 123, whereas experimental brain tumors in animals and tissue-cultured human gliomas and metastatic tumors accumulate the dye, with a maximum concentration being evident at 4 hours after intravenous administration.[9,105] Myocardium, choroid plexus, and the proximal convoluted tubule of the kidney also accumulate rhodamine 123.[68] Rhodamine 123 is tumoricidal in the presence of blue-green light, with an absorption maximum of 512 nm in a physiologic environment.[67] Preliminary laboratory findings suggest that phototoxic reaction produced with rhodamine 123 and light is tumor-cell specific, with injury primarily directed at the mitochondria of tumor cells.[70] Probably owing to the lipophilic property of rhodamine 123, tumor cells outside of the BBB demonstrate rhodamine 123 fluorescence[9] and would be expected to be photosensitive. Some tellurium, selenium, and sulfur pyrylium dyes that are also cationic share many of the tissue distribution characteristics of rhodamine 123 and thus may be shown to be effective photosensitizers.[70] The potential advantage of the pyrylium compounds lies in their ability to absorb light in the near-infrared spectrum between 700 and 850 nm wavelength, where there is little interference with light transmission by most biologic tissues. Theoretically, it would be possible to treat a larger volume of tissue with PCT using one of these compounds than is currently available with either rhodamine 123 or HPD. Without question, the limiting factor on the successful application of PCT for the treatment of malignant gliomas at present has been the lack of a tumor-specific photosensitizer that can be activated by light that is readily transmitted through brain.

LIGHT DOSIMETRY

Light transmission through tissue is determined by the optical characteristics of the tissue and the wavelength of light. Most tissues contain variable concentrations of biopigments that are primarily responsible for the absorption of visible light. Water, which accounts for approximately 60% to 70% of tissue by weight, readily absorbs ultraviolet and far-infrared light. Hemoglobin, melanin, and the cytochromes are the principle biopigments involved in the absorption of visible light. The penetrance distance is defined as the distance at which the light intensity has fallen to $1/e$ or 37% of its initial value. In cadaveric human brain, the light penetrance is 0.2 to 0.4 mm at 488 nm, 1.2 to 1.6 mm at 660 nm, and 1.5 to 1.7 mm at 710 nm.[105] In living rat brain, light from an intracerebral emitting point source is attenuated by 99% at a distance of 3.8 mm at 488 nm and at 4.9 mm at 633 nm.[106] The light is attenuated to a larger degree in the presence of a photosensitizer that absorbs light at the particular wavelength being studied.[106,107] This has been referred to as a shielding effect.[107] Tissue concentrations of HPD that are greater than 5 μg/mg significantly increase the attenuation coefficient to red light so that further increasing the tissue concentration of HPD actually decreases the photoreactive yield by preventing penetration of red light at depth.[107]

Metabolic activity also affects the transparency of biologic tissues to light.[108,109] Hypertonic solutions increase optical density, probably owing to changes in the shape and volume of erythrocytes secondary to changes in the plasma osmolarity.[110] Hypotonicity, which causes swelling of red blood cells, resulting in increased red blood cell surface area, will result in increased light transmission. Changes in the optical density of blood produced by changes in plasma osmolarity, in the rate of blood flow, and in blood PCO_2 may occur over a wide range of wavelengths. These physiologic changes may be associated with complex and oftentimes unpredictable changes in the light penetrance characteristics of tissue. Thus, experimental measurements of light penetration through tissues serve only as rough estimates of the actual penetration of a particular wavelength of light, particularly when applying this information for planning an effective light dose for PCT. It has been helpful to obtain dynamic real-time measurements of light intensity within tissue during PCT more clearly to understand the mechanism of tumor cell killing and better to plan light dosimetry for treatment.[106]

The most efficient excitation wavelength is that which corresponds to the maximum absorption wavelength of the photosensitizer. For HPD, maximum light absorption is seen with a wavelength between 400 and 410 nm; however, because of the poor tissue penetrability at shorter wavelengths, a wavelength of approximately 630 nm (red light) is used to excite the drug.[111] In vitro and in vivo studies indicate that the photosensitizing efficiency of HPD photodynamic therapy is not affected by nonthermal variations in dose rates of delivered light.[112] Photochemotherapeutic activity thus depends on the total dose of light that is delivered (total energy) and not the light fluency. Similar findings were reported with rhodamine 123, which demonstrated time-dependent tumoricidal activity in the presence of blue-green laser light that was independent of the rate of light delivery.[67] Continuous light delivery appears necessary for phototoxicity in that pulsed laser light is ineffective in activating HPD in vivo.[113]

Original studies used either a filtered or nonfiltered high-intensity white light source, such as a xenon arc lamp, to photoactivate HPD. Currently, lasers are

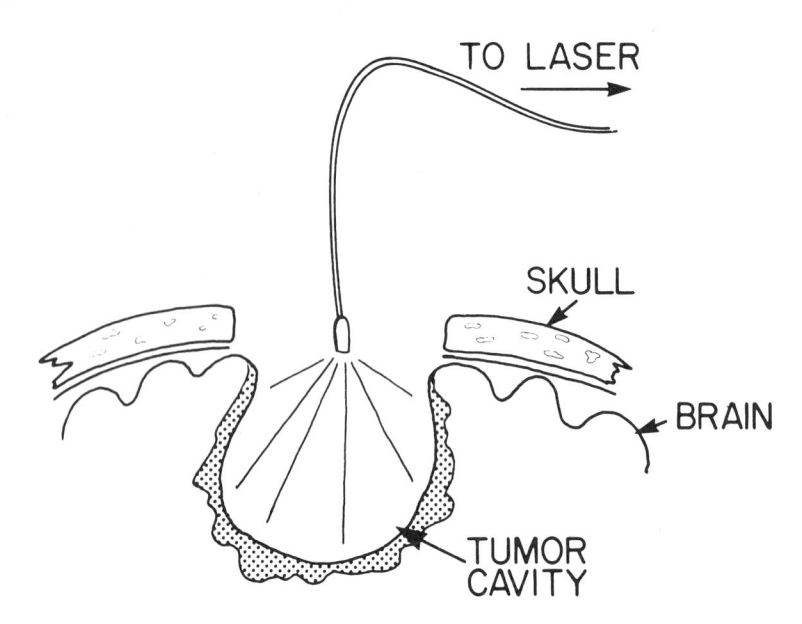

FIG 12–3.
Technique of surface illumination of tumor bed after tumor debulking.

used to produce high-intensity monochromatic light that is transmitted via a quartz fiberoptic cable to the tumor for treatment. The argon pumped dye laser, with rhodamine 590, kiton red, or (DCM) dye, produces red light with a wavelength of about 630 nm that is used to activate HPD. These systems have a maximum output of 1.5 to 2.0 W of red light. The gold vapor laser, which reportedly is capable of 5 to 10 W of red light output, is also under investigation.[56] The continuous-wave argon-ion laser, which is capable of 15 W of output measured at tissue, has been used for activation of rhodamine 123. Modifications in the argon pumped dye laser for use with infrared-emitting dyes are under investigation for use in PCT using the pyrylium dye compounds.

Several techniques have been employed for delivery of the laser light to the tumor. After gross tumor resection, laser light can be applied to the surface of the tumor cavity with either a divergent bare-tipped fiber[57] or microlens assembly (Fig 12–3). Special diffusing media have also been employed to help scatter the laser light to illuminate the tumor cavity more thoroughly with a single laser application.[114] A diffusion medium–filled balloon system into which the laser fiberoptic is placed has been devised by Muller and Wilson[55] (Fig 12–4). Smaller centrencephalic tumors are best treated by the stereotaxic interstitial placement of spherical or cylindrical emitting laser fiber tips (Fig12–5).

The rate of light delivery will be limited by nonspecific thermal effects of the laser that are associated with higher fluencies. Duration of light exposure will depend on the penetrability of the light, the depth of tissue that is to be treated, and the light fluency, assuming that phototoxicity is a function of total energy delivered.

THERMAL CONSIDERATIONS

Hematoporphyrin derivative phototherapy as previously reported by most clinicians has had at least a partially hyperthermic effect.[115,116] It is known that only mild temperature elevations (41 to 42°C) for a sustained time are selectively cytotoxic to cancer cells.[117-119] Increases in temperature are correlated with increases in light fluency, that is, the rate of light delivery. During light delivery at a constant power setting, the temperature will rapidly rise during the first 4 minutes of exposure to an equilibrium temperature.[115] Surface irradiation of the skin in mice with red light at 630 nm produces subcutaneous temperature ele-

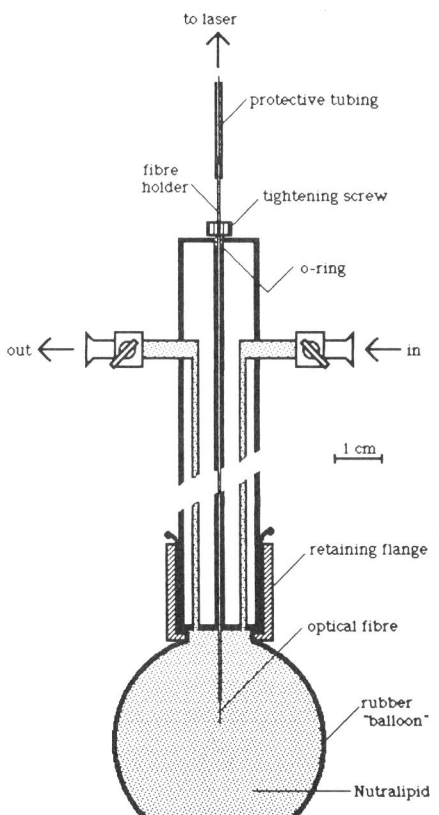

FIG 12-4.
Laser fiber-balloon irradiator. The balloon is placed into the tumor resection cavity and inflated to the volume of the tumor tissue removed with a light-scattering medium (Nutralipid). A bare-tipped, 400-μm-diameter quartz optical fiber is placed into the interior of the balloon and then coupled to a dye laser. Uniform surface irradiation of the tumor bed is accomplished with this technique. (Courtesy of Dr. Brian Wilson.)

TO LASER

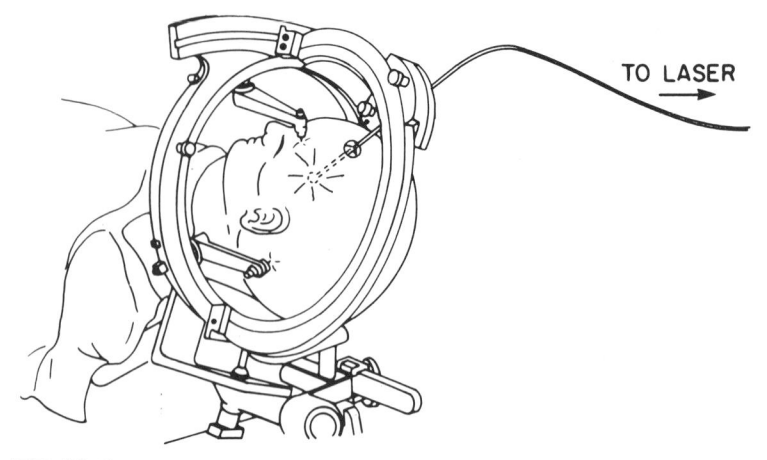

FIG 12-5.
Stereotaxis implantation of quartz fiberoptic laser light-emitting source.

vations of 4°C at 200 mW/sq cm, 6°C at 300 mW/sq cm, and 10°C at 400 mW/ sq cm.[112] Temperature rise is more significant during interstitial laser light application through an implanted fiberoptic. Kinsey et al.[115] recorded temperature measurements around a 400-μm quartz fiber tip that was implanted into the center of a subcutaneously implanted murine mammary tumor. They found a temperature rise of approximately 20°C at a power input of 200 mW/sq cm and of approximately 7°C at a power input of 100 mW/sq cm at a distance of 5 mm lateral to the fiber tip. Our laboratory has studied the thermal rise in normal rat brain in response to interstitial laser irradiation from both a bare-tipped and a diffusing sapphire - tipped quartz fiberoptic for both argon laser light (454 to 514.5 nm) and red light (630 nm) from an argon pumped dye laser with DCM dye. There is a much greater rise in tissue temperature, particularly near the fiberoptic tip for the bare-tipped fiber; this undoubtedly reflects the extremely high power density present at the tip of the bare fiber due to the smaller surface area of emission (Fig 12–6).

A synergistic interaction exists between PCT with HPD and hyperthermia (40.5 to 45°C).[120-123] The sensitizing effect of hyperthermia varies both with temperature and the sequence of heat treatment and PCT treatment. The greatest potentiation of PCT with HPD occurs when hyperthermia is administered immediately after PCT.[120,121,123] It has been suggested that hyperthermia inhibits repair of PCT-induced damage. The temperatures generated during standard PCT surface irradiation with 100 to 200 mW/sq cm do not appear to be high enough or long enough in duration to offer hyperthermic potentiation of PCT with HPD.[120] At longer light exposure times or higher power densities, there may be hyperthermic interaction present. Certainly based on the temperature data obtained from interstitial laser light delivery, hyperthermia would be expected to play some role in the tissue changes following PCT.

CLINICAL EXPERIENCE

Several medical centers are currently treating malignant brain tumors with PCT using HPD and red light. In the United States these are pilot clinical research projects designed to study the feasibility and potential efficacy of this form of treatment. At present, HPD is not available commercially for use in neurosurgical patients. Since research began in 1978, there have been just over 50 cases of PCT-treated brain tumor reported in the literature.[52-57]

Laws and Wharen[54] last reported a total clincial experience of 22 patients with malignant brain tumors (17 malignant gliomas, two metastases, two medulloblastomas, one rhabdomyosarcoma) in 1984. They were treating deep, surgically inaccessible solid or cystic tumors by stereotaxic implantation of a laser fiberoptic probe and irradiation without tumor removal 24 hours after intravenous administration of HPD. Other tumors were treated by tumor removal followed by irradiation of the tumor bed with either a high-intensity filtered white light source or broad-beam fiberoptic. Based on laboratory studies, they assumed a maximum depth or radius of tumor-cell kill of 8 mm using a power density of 25 mW/sq

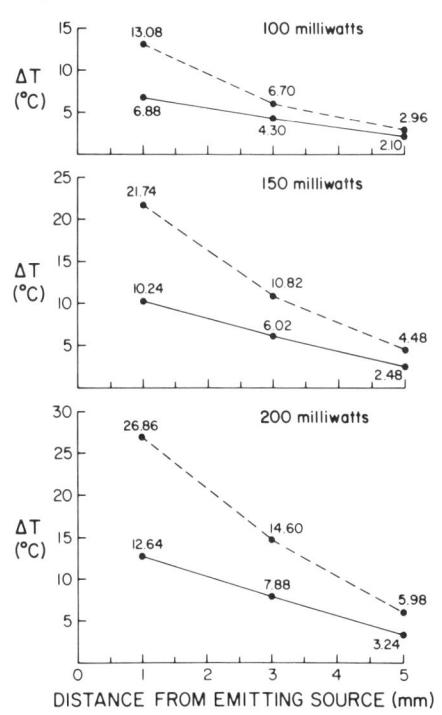

FIG 12-6.
Comparison of temperature rise (ΔT) in rat brain tissue adjacent to an intracerebral bare-tipped (*broken line*) and a frosted sapphire-tipped (*solid line*) quartz optical fiber. Laser light was generated by an argon laser, and power output was measured out of the end of each fiber. Note the very high (thermally damaging) temperatures generated by the unshielded bare-tipped fiber at distances less than 3 mm away for 150 and 200 mW of laser power.

cm and total dose of 160 J. In their series there were three postoperative infections, no deaths and two instances of postoperative cerebral edema related to the therapy. Hematoporphyrin-derivative was present in all of the tumor specimens removed, but the concentration varied.

Muller and Wilson[55] reported on eight patients with malignant primary brain tumor treated with PCT using HPD_1 and tumor cavity photoillumination with an inflatable balloon filled with a scattering medium into which was placed a fiberoptic coupled to an argon pumped dye laser. The total light energy delivered ranged from 8 to 68 J/sq cm. They had no adverse photosensitivity skin reactions and no cases of acute postoperative deterioration due to edema. Two patients developed wound infections; one required removal of an infected bone flap.

McCulloch et al.[56] reported on 16 patients with malignant tumors (nine glioblastomas, two oligodendrogliomas, one grade 2/3 astrocytoma, four metastases) treated with red light at 48 hours after intravenous HPD (5 mg/kg). Patients underwent standard neurosurgical treatment with craniotomy and radical tumor excision. Early in the series, red light was administered from either an argon pumped dye laser with rhodamine dye or from a special filtered incandescent lamp that was capable of a total output of 24 W in the spectral range between 620 and 720 nm. Recently, a gold vapor laser with an output of 1.5 W at 627.8 nm has been used. All patients with malignant gliomas were also treated with 5,000 rad of whole-brain irradiation. Cerebral edema was present in nearly all cases after treatment. Mannitol and steroids were necessary to treat many of these cases. Of three patients with limited tumor resection, two had an increase in their postoperative neurologic deficit and one died of severe cerebral edema. Photosensitivity of the skin occurred in some of the patients, in whom precautionary measures were inadequate.

The earliest report using HPD PCT was by Perria et al. in 1980.[53] They treated nine patients with various types of malignant brain tumors using a dose of HPD between 2.5 and 10.0 mg/kg body weight and a light dosage of 9 J/sq cm from a helium-neon laser. They, like every other investigator to date, were unable to show any real benefit from the treatment.

The most common complication of PCT with HPD is skin sensitivity to sunlight or intense artificial light. In patients who are exposed to bright light, pain, swelling, and rash may result for up to 4 weeks after the injection of HPD. As a consequence, these patients must be kept isolated from potentially harmful light exposure. In addition, the scalp and meninges, since they contain high levels of HPD, must be protected from light exposure during the irradiation process in PCT. As mentioned above, cerebral edema is commonly noted after PCT with HPD and can lead to secondary brain injury. The edema may represent brain response to vascular injury induced by PCT or hyperthermic injury resulting from too rapid a rate of light delivery. Steroids appear to offer protection against development of edema following PCT.[54]

FUTURE CONSIDERATIONS

The use of PCT in treating brain tumors is still in its infancy. Difficulties found with the use of HPD indicate that more tumor-specific agents are needed. Ideally, the photosensitizer should bind only to tumor cells, whatever their location, and have little to no affinity for normal tissues either adjacent to the tumor or elsewhere in the body. The photosensitizer should absorb light in the spectral range that readily penetrates tissue (near-infrared) and be converted into a tumoricidal intermediate that efficiently kills tumor cells. Such an agent has yet to be discovered. Work is under way exploring the possibility of binding photosensitizers such as hematoporphyrin to tumor-specific antibodies as a means of increasing therapeutic specificity.[124] Preliminary studies have also focused on the use of mitochondrial-specific dyes, pyryliums, that have an affinity for transformed cell lines and absorb light in the near-infrared spectrum. Further investigations will follow aimed at maximizing the intratumoral concentration of the drug and decreasing its systemic effects.

Should an infrared-absorbing tumor-specific dye be found, it will require a light source capable of high-intensity outputs over its spectral range of absorption. The production of infrared-producing dye lasers and improvements in diode (gallium arsenide) lasers that emit in the near-infrared range may be the answer.

Lastly, the issue remains unresolved regarding the mechanism of PCT-induced tumoricidal activity. Clearly this will depend on the photosensitizer and the wavelength of light employed. An understanding of the nature of tumor-specific binding of an ideal photosensitizer will come when we understand the property that is commonly shared by cancer cells and distinguishes them from normal cells or it will come by serendipity.

REFERENCES

1. Raab O: Uber die kinkung fluoresciren der stoff auf infusoniera. *Z Biol* 1900; 39:524.
2. Dougherty TJ: Activated dyes as antitumor agents. *JNCI* 1974; 52:1333–1336.
3. Rall DP, Loo TL, Lane M, et al: Appearance and persistence of fluorescent material in tumor tissue after tetracycline administration. *JNCI* 1957; 19:79–85.
4. Duran-Reynals F: Studies on the localization of dyes and foreign proteins in normal and malignant tissues. *Am J Cancer* 1939; 35:98–107.
5. Rasmussen-Taxdal DS, Ward GE, Figge FHJ: Fluorescence of human lymphatic and cancer tissues following high doses of intravenous hematoporphyrin. *Cancer* 1955; 8:78–81.
6. Moore GE: Fluorescein as an agent in the differentiation of normal and malignant tissues. *Science* 1947; 106:130–131.
7. Wilbanks GD, Richart RM: Fluorescence of cervical intraepithelial neoplasia induced by tetracycline and acridine orange. *Am J Obstet Gynecol* 1970; 106:726–730.
8. Mellors RC, Glassman A, Papanicolaou GN: A microfluorimetric scanning method for the detection of cancer cells in smears of exfoliated cells. *Cancer* 1952; 5:458–468.

9. Beckman WC, Powers SK, Brown JT: Differential retention of rhodamine 123 by avian sarcoma virus induced glioma and normal brain tissue of the rat. *Cancer*, submitted for publication.
10. Ben-Hur E, Rosenthal I: Photosensitized inactivation of Chinese hamster cells by phthalocyanines. *Photochem Photobiol* 1985; 42:129–133.
11. Auler H, Banzer G: Untersuchungen uber die rolle der prophine bei geschwulstkranken menschen and tieren. *Z Krebsforsch* 1942; 53:65–68.
12. Figge FHJ, Weiland GS, Manganiello LOJ: Cancer detection and therapy: Affinity of neoplastic, embryonic, and traumatized tissues for porphyrins and metalloporphyrins. *Proc Soc Exp Biol Med* 1948; 68:640–641.
13. Lipson RL, Baldes EJ, Olsen AM: The use of a derivative of hematoporphyrin in tumor detection. *JNCI* 1961; 26:1–11.
14. Lipson RL, Baldes EJ, Olsen AM: Hematoporphyrin derivative: A new aid for endoscopic detection of malignant disease. *J Thorac Cardiovasc Surg*, 1961; 42:623–641.
15. Lipson RL, Baldes EJ, Olsen AM: Further evaluation of the use of hematoporphyrin derivative as a new aid for the endoscopic detection of malignant disease. *Disease Chem*, 1964; 46:676–679.
16. Lipson RL, Pratt JH, Baldes EJ, et al: Hematoporphyrin derivative for detection of cervical cancer. *Obstet Gynecol* 1964; 24:78–84.
17. Lipson RL, Gray MJ, Baldes EJ: Hematoporphyrin derivative for detection and management of cancer. *Proceedings of the Ninth International Cancer Congress*. 1966; p. 393.
18. Diamond I, Granelli SG, McDonagh AF, et al: Photodynamic therapy of malignant tumours. *Lancet* 1972; 2:1175–1177.
19. Star WM, Marijnissen JPA, Vanden Berg-Blok AE, et al: Destructive effect of photoradiation on the microcirculation of a rat mammary tumor growing in "sandwich" observation chambers, in Doiron DR, Gomer CJ (eds): *Porphyrin Localization and Treatment of Tumors*. New York, Alan R Liss, 1984, pp 637–645.
20. Henderson BW, Dougherty TJ, Malone PB: Studies on the mechanism of tumor destruction by photoradiation therapy, in Doiron DR, Gomer CJ (eds): *Porphyrin Localization and Treatment of Tumors*, New York, Alan R. Liss, 1984, pp 601–612.
22. Gomer CJ, Jester JV, Razum NJ, et al: Photodynamic therapy of intraocular tumors: Examination of hematoporphyrin derivative distribution and longterm damage in rabbit occular tissue. *Cancer Res* 1985; 45:3718–3725.
23. Perlin DS, Murant RS, Gibson SL, et al: Effects of photosensitization by hematoporphyrin derivative on mitochondrial adenosine triphosphatase-mediated proton transport and membrane integrity of R3230AC mammary adenocarcinoma. *Cancer Res* 1985; 45:653.
24. Henderson BW, Waldow SM, Mang TS, et al: Tumor destruction and kinetics of tumor cell death in two experimental mouse tumors following photodynamic therapy. *Cancer Res* 1985; 45:572–576.
25. Dougherty TJ, Grindey GB, Fiel R, et al: Photoradiation therapy: II. Cure of animal tumors with hematoporphyrin and light. *JNCI* 1975; 55:115–121.
26. McPhee MS, Thorndyke CW, Thomas G, et al: Interstitial applications of laser irradiation in hematoporphyrin derivative-photosensitized Dunning R3327 prostate cancers. *Lasers Surg Med* 1984; 4:93–98.
27. Dougherty TJ, Thoma RE, Boyle DG, et al: Interstitial photoradiation therapy for primary solid tumors in pet cats and dogs. *Cancer Res* 1981; 41:401–404.

28. Berenbaum MC, Bonnett R, Scourides PA: In vivo biological activity of the components of hematoporphyrin derivative. *Br J Cancer* 1982; 45:571–581.
29. Nseyo UO, Dougherty TJ, Boyle D, et al: Experimental photodynamic treatment of canine bladder. *J Urol* 1985; 133:311–315.
30. Selman SH, Milligan AJ, Kreimer-Brinbaum M, et al: Hematoporphyrin derivative photochemotherapy of experimental bladder tumors. *J Urol* 1985; 133:330–333.
31. Bellnier DA, Prout GR, Lin CW: Effect of 514.5-nm argon ion laser radiation on hematoporphyrin derivative-treated bladder tumor cells in vitro and in vivo. *JNCI* 1985; 74:617–625.
32. Cowled PA, Forbes IJ: Photocytotoxicity in vivo of haematoporphyrin derivative components. *Cancer Lett* 1985; 28:111–118.
33. Shikowitz MJ, Steinberg BM, Abramson AL: Hematoporphyrin derivative therapy of papillomas. *Arch Otolaryngol Head Neck Surg* 1986; 112:42–46.
34. Dougherty TJ, Lawrence G, Kaufman JH, et al: Photoradiation in the treatment of recurrent breast carcinoma. *JNCI* 1979; 62:231–237.
35. Hayata Y, Kato H, Konaka C, et al: Fiberoptic bronchoscopic laser photoradiation for tumor localization in lung cancer. *Chest* 1982; 82:10–14.
36. Cortese DA, Kinsey JH: Endoscopic management of lung cancer with hematoporphyrin derivative phototherapy. *Mayo Clin Proc* 1982; 57:543–547.
37. Wile AG, Dahlman A, Burns RG, et al: Laser photoradiation therapy of cancer following hematoporphyrin sensitization. *Lasers Surg Med* 1982; 2:163–168.
38. Forbes IJ, Cowled PA, Leong ASY, et al: Phototherapy of human tumours using haematoporphyrin derivative. *Med J Aust* 1980; 2:489–493.
39. McCaughan JS: Photoradiation of malignant tumors presensitized with hematoporphyrin derivative, in Doiron DR, Gomer CJ (eds): *Porphyrin Localization and Treatment of Tumors,* New York, Alan R Liss, Inc., 1984, pp 805–827.
40. Forbes IJ, Ward AD, Jacka FJ, et al: Multidisciplinary approach to phototherapy of human cancers, in Doiron DR, Gomer CJ (eds): *Porphyrin Localization and Treatment of Tumors,* New York, Alan R Liss. 1984, pp 693–708.
41. Schuller DE, McCaughan JS Rock RP: Photodynamic therapy in head and neck cancer. *Arch Otolaryngol Head Neck Surg* 1985; 111:351–355.
42. Wile AG, Novotny J, Mason R., et al: Photoradiation therapy of head and neck cancer, in Doiron DR, Gomer CJ (eds): *Porphyrin Localization and Treatment of Tumors.* New York, Alan R Liss, 1984, pp 681–691.
43. Balchum OJ. Doiron DR, Huth GC: HpD photodynamic therapy for obstructing lung cancer, in Doiron DR, Gomer CJ (eds): *Porphyrin Localization and Treatment of Tumors.* New York, Alan R Liss, 1984, pp 727–745.
44. Bruce RA: Photoradiation of choroidal malignant melanoma, in Doiron DR, Gomer CJ (eds): *Porphyrin Localization and Treatment of Tumors.* New York, Alan R Liss, 1984, pp 777–784.
45. Misaki T, Hisazumi H, Miyoshi N: *Photoradiation Therapy of Bladder Tumors.* New York, Alan R Liss, 1984, pp 785–794.
46. Tomio L, Calzavara F, Zorat PL, et al: Photoradiation therapy for cutaneous and subcutaneous malignant tumors using hematoporphyrin, in Doiron DR, Gomer CJ (eds): *Porphyrin Localization and Treatment of Tumors.* New York, Alan R Liss, 1984, pp 829–840.
47. Hayata Y, Kato H, Okitsu H, et al: Photodynamic therapy with hematoporphyrin derivative in cancer of the upper gastrointestinal tract. *Semin Surg Oncol* 1985; 1:1–11.

48. Nseyo UO, Dougherty TJ, Boyle DG, et al: Whole bladder photodynamic therapy for transitional cell carcinoma of bladder. *Urology* 1985; 26:274–280.
49. Hayata Y, Kato H, Konaka C, et al: Hematoporphyrin derivative and photoradiation therapy in early stage lung cancer. *Lasers Surg Med* 1984; 4:39–47.
50. Benson RC: Endoscopic management of bladder cancer with hematoporphyrin derivative phototherapy. *Urol Clin North Am* 1984; 11:637–642.
51. Bruce RA: Evaluation of hematoporphyrin photoradiation therapy to treat choroidal melanomas. *Lasers Surg Med* 1984; 4:59–64.
52. Forbes IJ: Photochemotherapy of human cancers with hematoporphyrin derivative. *Med J Aust* 1984; 140:94–96.
53. Perria C, Capuzzo T, Cavagnaro G, et al: First attempts at the photodynamic treatment of human gliomas. *J Neurosurg Sci,* 1980; 24:119–129.
54. Laws ER, Wharen RE: Comment effects of photoradiation therapy on normal rat brain. *Neurosurgery* 1984; 15:808–809.
55. Muller PJ Wilson BC: Photodynamic therapy: Cavitary photoillumination of malignant cerebral tumors using a laser coupled inflatable balloon. *Can J Neurol Sci* 1985; 12:371–373.
56. McCulloch GAJ, Forbes IJ, See KL, et al: Phototherapy in malignant brain tumors, in Doiron DR, Gomer CJ (eds): *Porphyrin Localization and Treatment of Tumors.* New York, Alan R Liss, 1984, pp 709–717.
57. Laws ER, Cortese DA, Kinsey JH, et al: Photoradiation therapy in the treatment of malignant brain tumors: A phase I (feasibility) study. *Neurosurgery* 1981; 9:672–678.
58. Cheng MK, McKean J, Boivert D, et al: Effects of photoradiation therapy on normal rat brain. *Neurosurgery* 1984; 15:804–810.
59. Boggan JE, Walter R, Edwards MSB, et al: Distribution of hematoporphyrin derivative in the rat 9L gliosarcoma brain tumor analyzed by digital video fluorescence microscopy. *J Neurosurg* 1984; 61:1113–1119.
60. Little FM, Gomer CJ, Hyman S, et al: Observation in studies of quantitative kinetics of tritium labelled hematoporphyrin derivatives (HpD_I and HpD_{II}) in the normal and neoplastic rat brain model. *J. Neurooncol* 1984; 2:361–370.
61. Wharen RE, Anderson RE, Laws ER: Quantitation of hematoporphyrin derivative in human gliomas, experimental central nervous system tumors, and normal tissues. *Neurosurgery* 1983; 12:446–450.
62. Boisvert DPJ, McKean JDS, Tulip J, et al: Penetration of hematoporphyrin derivative into rat brain and intracerebral 9L glioma tissue. *J. Neurooncol* 1985; 3:113–118.
63. Boggan JE, Bolger C, Edwards MSB: Effect of hematoporphyrin derivative photoradiation therapy on survival in the rat 9L gliosarcoma brain-tumor model. *J. Neurosurg* 1985; 63:917–921.
64. Kaye AH, Morstyn G, Ashcraft RG: Uptake and retention of hematoporphyrin derivative in an in vivo/in vitro model of cerebral glioma. *Neurosurgery* 1985; 17:883–890.
65. Boggan JE, Edwards MSB, Berns MW, et al: Hematoporphyrin derivative photoradiation therapy of the rat 9L gliosarcoma brain tumor model. *Lasers Surg Med* 1984; 4:99–105.
66. Cheng MK, McKean J, Mielke B, et al: Photoradiation therapy of 9L-gliosarcoma in rats: Hematoporphyrin derivative (types I and iI) followed by laser energy. *J Neurooncol* 1985; 3:217–228.
67. Powers SK, Pribil S, Gillespie GY, et al: Laser photochemotherapy of rhodamine-123 sensitized human glioma cells in vitro. *J Neurosurg* 1986; 64:918–923.

68. Banes AJ, Link GW, Beckman WC, et al: HPLC quantitation of rhodamines 123 and 110 from tissues and cultured cells. *J Chromatogr* 1986; 356:301–309.
69. Edwards MSB: Photosensitization of malignant glioma cells with acridine orange. *Sixth International Conference on Brain Tumor Research and Therapy.* 1985.
70. Powers SK: Photochemotherapy with cationic lipophilic dye compounds. *Sixth International Conference on Brain Tumor Research and Therapy.* 1985.
71. Wrenn FR, Good ML, Handler, P: The use of positron-emitting radioisotopes for the localization of brain tumors. *Science* 1951; 113:525–527.
72. Frigerio NA: US Patent 307391, 1962.
73. Ben-Hur E, Carmichael A, Riesz P, et al: Photochemical generation of superoxide radical and the cytotoxicity of phthalocyanines. *Int J Radiat Biol* 1985; 48:837–846.
74. Dougherty TJ, Potter WR, Weishaupt KR: The structure of the active component of hematoporphyrin derivative, in Doiron DR, Gomer CJ (eds): *Porphyrin Localization and Treatment of Tumors.* New York, Alan R Liss, 1984, pp 301–314.
75. Dougherty TJ, Boyle DG, Weishaupt KR, et al: Photoradiation therapy: Clinical and drug advances, in Kessel D, Dougherty TJ (eds): *Porphyrin Photosensitization.* New York, Plenum Publishing Corp, 1983, p 3.
76. Moan J, Christensen T, Sommer S: The main photosensitizing components of hematoporphyrin derivative. *Cancer Lett* 1982; 15:161–166.
77. Spikes JD: Photobiology of porphyrins, in Doiron DR, Gomer CJ (eds) *Porphyrin Localization and Treatment of Tumors.* New York, Alan R Liss, 1984, pp 19–39.
78. Kessel D: Hematoporphyrin and HpD: Photophysics, photochemistry and phototherapy. *Photochem Photobiol* 1984; 39:851–859.
79. Sandberg S, Romslo I, Hovding G, et al: Porphyrin-induced photodamage as related to the subcellular localization of the porphyrins. *Acta Dermatol Suppl* 1982; 100:75–80.
80. Denstman SC, Dillehay LE, Williams JR: Enhanced susceptibility to HpD-sensitized phototoxicity and correlated resistance to trypsin detachment in SV40 transformed IMR-90 cells. *Photochem Photobiol* 1986; 43:145–147.
81. Kochevar IE: Photoxicity mechanisms: Chlorpromozine photosensitized damage to DNA and cell membranes. *J Invest Dermatol* 1981; 76:59–64.
82. Dubbelman TMAR, DeGoeij AFPM, Van Stevenick J: Protoporphyrin-induced photodynamic effects on transport processes across the membrane of human erythrocytes. *Acta Biochim Biophys Acad Sci Hung* 1980; 595:133–139.
83. Girotti AW: Photodynamic action of protoporphyrin IX on human erythrocytes: Cross-linking of membrane proteins. *Biochem Biophys Res Commun* 1976; 72:1367–1374.
84. Moan J, Steen HB, Feren K, et al: Uptake of hematoporphyrin derivative and sensitized photoinactivation of C3H cells with different oncogenic potential. *Cancer Lett* 1981; 14:291–296.
85. Salzberg S, Lejbkowics F, Ehrenberg B, et al: Protective effect of cholesterol on Friend leukemic cells against photosensitization by hematoporphyrin derivative. *Cancer Res* 1985; 45:3305–3310.
86. Shulok JR, Klaunig JE, Selman SH, et al: Cellular effects of hematoporphyrin derivative photodynamic therapy on normal and neoplastic rat bladder cells. *Am J Pathol* 1986; 122:277–283.
87. Hull DS, Green K, Hampstead D: Effect of hematoporphyrin derivative on rabbit corneal epithelial cell function and ultrastructure. *Invest Ophthalmol Vis Sci* 1985; 26:1465–1474.

88. Coppola A, Viggiani E, Salzarulo L, et al: Ultrastructural changes in lymphoma cells treated with hematoporphyrin and light. *Am J Pathol* 1980; 99:175–192.
89. Berns MW, Dhalman A, Johnson FM, et al: In vitro cellular effects of hematoporphyrin derivative. *Cancer Res* 42:2325–2329, 1982.
90. Sandberg S: Protoporphyrin-induced photodamage to mitochondria and lysosomes from rat liver. *Clin Chem Acta* 1981; 111:55.
91. Evensen JF, Moan J: Photodynamic actions and chromosomal damage: A comparison of haematoporphyrin derivative (HpD) and light. *Br J Cancer* 1982; 45:456.
92. Mitchell JB, McPherson S, Degraff W, et al: Oxygen dependance of hematoporphyrin derivative-induced photoinactivation of Chinese hamster cells. *Cancer Res* 1985; 45:2008–2011.
93. See KL, Forbes IJ, Betts WH: Oxygen dependency of photocytotoxicity with hematoporphyrin derivative. *Photochem Photobiol* 1984; 39:631.
94. Bugelski PJ, Porter CW, Dougherty TJ: Autoradiographic distribution of hematoporphyrin derivative in normal and tumor tissue of the mouse. *Cancer Res* 1981; 41:4606–4612.
95. Wise BL, Taxdal DR: Studies of the blood-brain barrier utilizing hematoporphyrin. *Brain Res* 1967; 4:387–389.
96. Winkelman J, Rasmussen-Taxdal DS: Quantitative determination of porphyrin uptake by tumor tissue following parenteral administration. *Bull Johns Hopkins Hosp* 1960; 107:228–233.
97. Henderson BW, Waldwow SM, Marg TS, et al: Tumor destruction and kinetics of tumor cell death in two experimental mouse tumors following photodynamic therapy. *Cancer Res* 1985; 45:572–576.
98. Rounds DE, Doiron DR, Jacques DB, et al: Phototoxicity of brain tissue in hematoporphyrin derivative treated mice, in Doiron DR, Gomer CJ (eds): *Porphyrin Localization and Treatment of Tumors*. New York, Alan R Liss, 1984, pp 613–623.
99. Johnson LV, Walsh ML, Chen LB: Localization of mitochondria in living cells with rhodamine 123. *Proc Natl Acad Sci USA* 1980; 77:990–994.
100. Bernal SD, Lampidis TJ, Summerhayes IC, et al: Rhodamine 123 selectively reduces clonal growth of carcinoma cells in vitro. *Science* 1982; 218:1117–1119.
101. Johnson LV, Walsh MC, Bockus BJ, et al: Monitoring of relative mitochondrial membrane potential in living cells by fluorescence microscopy. *J. Cell Biol.* 1981; 88:526–535.
102. Lampidis TJ, Bernal SD, Summerhayes IC, et al: Selective toxicity of rhodamine 123 in carcinoma cells in vitro. *Cancer Res* 1983; 43:716–720.
103. Summerhayes IC, Lampidis TJ, Bernal SD, et al: Unusual retention of rhodamine 123 by mitochondria in muscle and carcinoma cells. *Proc Natl Acad Sci USA* 1982; 79:5292–5296.
104. Beckman WC, Powers SK: Differential retention of rhodamine 123 by normal brain and brain tumors from man in tissue culture. Submitted for publication.
105. Svasand LO, Ellinger R: Optical properties of human brain. *Photochem Photobiol* 1983; 38:293–299.
106. Powers SK, Brown JT: Light dosimetry in brain tissue: An in vivo model applicable to photodynamic therapy. *Lasers Surg Med* 1986; 6.
107. Doiron DR, Svassand LO, Profio AE: Light dosimetry in tissue: Application to photoradiation therapy. *Adv Exp Med Biol* 1981; 160:63–76.
108. Cummins JT, Pfeiffer E, Bright J: Measurements of light scattering changes in isolated tissues. *Anal Biochem* 1973; 56:264–269.

109. Jobsis FF: Noninvasive, infrared monitoring of cerebral and myocardial oxygen efficiency and circulatory parameters. *Science* 1977; 198:1264–1266.
110. Sinclair JD, Setterer WF, Fox IJ, et al: Apparent dye-dilution curves produced by injection of transparent solutions. *J Appl Physiol* 1961; 16:669–673.
111. Van Gemert JC, Berenbaum MC, Gijsbers GHM: Wavelength and light-dose dependence in tumor phototherapy with haematoporphyrin derivative. *Br J Cancer* 1985; 52:43–49.
112. Gomer CJ, Rucker, N, Razum NJ, et al: In vitro and in vivo light dose rate effects related to hematoporphyrin derivative photodynamic therapy. *Cancer Res* 1985; 45:1973–1977.
113. Bellnier DA, Lin CW, Parrish JA, et al: Hematoporphyrin derivative and pulse laser irradiation in Doiron DR, Gomer CJ (eds): *Porphyrin Localization and Treatment of Tumors*. New York, Alan R Liss, 1984, pp 533–540.
114. Jocham D, Staehler G, Chaussy C, et al: Integral dye-laser irradiation of photosensitized bladder tumors with the aid of a light-scattering medium, in Doiron DR, Gomer CJ (eds: *Porphyrin Localization and Treatment of Tumors*. New York, Alan R Liss, 1984, pp 249–256.
115. Kinsey JH, Cortese DA, Neel HB: Thermal considerations in murine tumor killing using hematoporphyrin derivative phototherapy. *Cancer Res* 1983; 43:1562–1567.
116. Svaasand LO, Doiron DR, Dougherty TJ: Temperature rise during photoradiation therapy of malignant tumors. *Med Phys* 1983; 10:10.
117. Mondovi B, Stom R, Rotilio G, et al: The biochemical mechanism of selective heat sensitivity of cancer cells: I. Studies on cellular respiration. *Cancer* 1969; 5:129–136.
118. Overgaard J: Effect of hyperthermia on malignant cells in vivo: A review and a hypothesis. *Cancer* 1977; 39:2637–2646.
119. Turano C, Ferraro A, Strom R, et al: The biochemical mechanism of selective heat sensitivity of cancer cells: III. Studies of lysosomes. *Cancer* 1970; 6:67–72.
120. Christensen T, Wahl A, Smedshammer L: Effects of haematoporphyrin derivative and light in combination with hyperthermia on cells in culture. *Br J Cancer* 1984; 50:85–89.
121. Waldow SM, Henderson BW, Dougherty TJ: Potentiation of photodynamic therapy by heat: Effect of sequence and time interval between treatment in vivo. *Lasers Surg Med* 1985; 5:83–94.
122. Waldow SM, Henderson BW, Dougherty TJ: Enhanced tumor control following sequential treatments of photodynamic therapy (PDT) and localized microwave hyperthermia in vivo. *Lasers Surg Med* 1984; 4:79–85.
123. Mang TS, Dougherty TJ: Time and sequence dependent influence of in vitro photodynamic therapy (PDT) survival by hyperthermia. *Photochem Photobiol* 1985; 42:533–540.
124. Mew D, Lum V, Wat CK, et al: Ability of specific monoclonal antibodies and conventional antisera conjugated to hematoporphyrin to label and kill selected cell lines subsequent to light activation. *Cancer Res* 1985: 45: 4380–4386.

13 Photoradiation Therapy of Malignant Brain Tumors

ROBERT E. WHAREN, JR., M.D.
ROBERT E. ANDERSON, B.S.
EDWARD R. LAWS, JR., M.D.

The concept of photoradiation therapy (PRT) is based on the ability of certain substances known as photosensitizers to concentrate preferentially in malignant tissue. These photosensitizers then have the capability to selectively destroy malignant tissue when activated by light of the appropriate wavelength and intensity in the presence of oxygen.

The action of a photosensitizer is produced by the absorption of photons of a wavelength sufficient to promote electrons within the sensitizer to an excited triplet state. This excited molecule may then interact either directly with substrates within the cell or indirectly with those substrates through the production of singlet oxygen. The various photochemical reactions that are excited by light are subsequently capable of killing cells through multiple interactions with the cell membrane, cytoplasm, nuclear membrane, and nucleus. In vivo, a major reaction is destruction of the tumor vasculature through damage to the endothelium.

An ideal photosensitizer should have a number of properties: (1) it should be selectively absorbed or retained by all neoplastic or dysplastic cells; (2) it must be efficient in killing malignant cells following application of light at a wavelength capable of significant tissue penetration; (3) it must be nontoxic to normal tissue; and (4) it should have some characteristic, such as fluorescence, that makes it easily detectable.

The search for an ideal photosensitizer is currently being pursued. Although far from ideal, the photosensitizer that has received the most extensive investigation in both the laboratory and the clinic is hematoporphyrin derivative (HPD).

Hematorporphyrin is a naturally occurring compound similar to the heme of hemoglobin without the iron ligand (Fig 13–1). Since the observation by Lipson et al. in 1960[31-33] that a derivative of hematoporphyrin (HPD) had superior tumor-localizing characteristics when compared with hematoporphyrin, all subsequent clinical studies have used HPD.

The first application of hematoporphyrin to the management of brain tumors took place in the 1950s at Johns Hopkins University, Baltimore.[39] A series of experiments were performed to evaluate hematoporphyrin fluorescence for the detection of brain tumors at the time of surgery. In this report, a patient with an olfactory-groove meningioma received 500 mg of hematoporphyrin intravenously 12 hours before surgery. At surgery, the tumor was observed to fluoresce

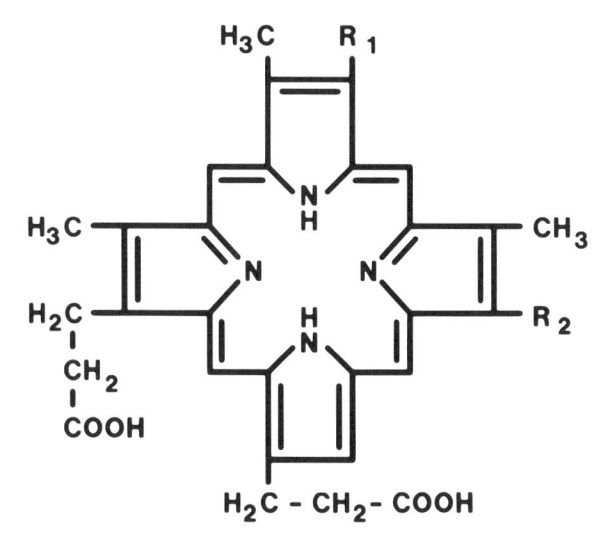

FIG 13-1.
The structure of hematoporphyrin. (From Laws ER, Cortese DA, Kinsey JH, et al: Photoradiation therapy in the treatment of malignant brain tumors: A phase I (feasibility) study. *Neurosurgery* 1981; 9:672–678. Used by permission.)

a brilliant red color. In addition, however, they described a patient with an ependymoma of the cervical cord who received 500 mg of hematoporphyrin, but in this case no fluorescence was observed.

Despite the use of HPD for the detection of malignant neoplasm, the first studies to suggest that photoactivation of hematoporphyrin might be cytotoxic to brain tumors were by Diamond et al. in 1972.[10] Using a glioma tumor model induced by methylnitrosourea in rats, they found that hematoporphyrin photoactivated by white light from fluorescent lamps was cytotoxic to glioma cells both in vitro and in vivo. Systemic hematoporphyrin caused extensive tumor necrosis in subcutaneously implanted gliomas when exposed to light, whereas neither light alone nor hematoporphyrin alone had any effect.

Dougherty et al. in 1975[15] described instances of eradication of experimental tumors using HPD and red light. Red light delivered 24 hours after drug administration prevented recurrences for at least 90 days in nearly half of a group of mice with subcutaneous mammary tumors. The use of red light at 630 nm provided much better tissue penetration when compared with violet light and resulted in a useful degree of tumor destruction.

The first reports of HPD photoradiation of human tumors appeared in 1976[16] and 1979[17] when Dougherty and coworkers found that cutaneous metastases of breast cancer and malignant melanoma could be selectively abated by PRT with HPD and red light. Since these initial reports, the concepts of HPD PRT have been applied to the treatment of a number of malignant neoplasms, including lung cancer,[8,12,13] bladder cancer,[2,24,26] head and neck tumors,[5,9,49,50] ocular tumors,[44] and brain tumors[20,29,34,36,37,45-47] with some success. The report by Hayata et al.[23] of the primary treatment of bronchial carcinoma with complete removal of small early lesions and a 3-year tumor-free survival is very encouraging and has been confirmed by Doiron.[12]

The application of PRT in neurosurgery was initially very encouraging. A number of investigators have reported the capability of HPD selectively to kill glioma cells both in vitro[10,21,48] and in vivo,[7,10,20,21,29,34,36,37] More recent reports have described initial attempts in the use of PRT for the treatment of malignant brain tumors.[20,29,34,36,37,45,47] Although the results are equivocal, it is evident that, despite major differences in the protocols by various investigators, HPD PRT is capable of tumor cell destruction in man. Rounds, et al.[40] and others,[3,6] however, have warned that hematoporphyrin is not entirely contained within neoplastic tissue and that some HPD accumulates in the brain tissue. This small amount of HPD within normal brain tissue can produce significant morbidity and mortality in experimental animals on application of a sufficient dose of light. The challenge is thus to determine parameters that produce effective cytotoxicity while minimizing any effect on normal brain.

LABORATORY INVESTIGATIONS

Laboratory efforts have been directed toward the goal of being able to take a biopsy from a patient and then to rapidly quantitate the amount of HPD in the tissue. If the amount of light necessary to produce a given volume of tumor destruction at a known concentration of HPD had been previously determined, then the nomogram would be available to determine the duration of light exposure necessary for a patient at the time of surgery. For this to be achieved, however, a number of questions had to be answered. It was first necessary to develop a method that could quantitate the amount of HPD rapidly in biopsy specimens. Previous methods of quantitating HPD have involved extraction techniques that are laborious and not readily applicable for a rapid determination in biopsy specimens. Further efforts were directed toward determining whether HPD concentrated exclusively within tumors or whether some HPD was present in normal brain. Efforts were directed toward determining the most efficient parameters of light application for brain tumors. Studies of the drug-light interaction and the time course of HPD absorption by brain tumors were performed in an effort to maximize the parameters of PRT. In addition, investigations of the mechanisms of cytotoxicity were done to determine whether HPD PRT could be effective in hypoxic tissue, as many malignant brain tumors contain hypoxic or necrotic regions within the tumor.

The assay system developed[45] was a microfluorescence assay in which the tissue sample is frozen in a cryostat and the surface is sectioned flat. The sample is then subjected to fluorescence microscopy, which quantitates the fluorescence from an 80 μ diameter region of tissue. The HPD concentration is obtained from a calibration curve (Fig 13–2). This microfluorescence assay system proved to be reliable for quantitation of HPD in brain tissue when compared with quantitation of HPD using a tritiated radioactive label.

Quantitation of HPD in experimental tumors induced in rats using ethylnitrosourea (Table 13–1) revealed levels of approximately 1 μg of HPD per gram of tissue 24 hours following the administration of 5 mg/kg of HPD.[45] At 4 hours after HPD administration, there was approximately 12 μg of HPD per gram of tissue. In comparison with the tumor, the normal brain had HPD levels of 0.6

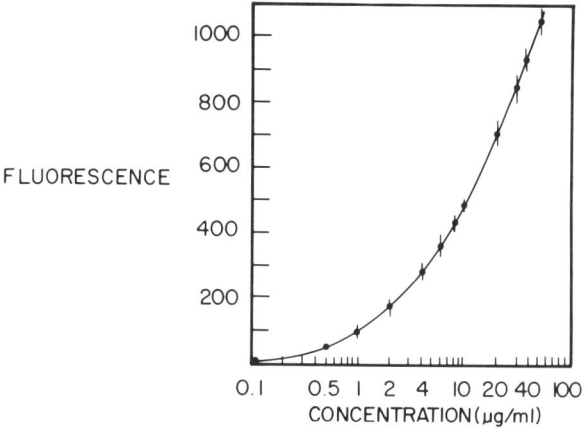

FIG 13–2.
Calibration curve of intensity of fluorescence vs. concentration of hematoporphyrin derivative in 9.9% sodium chloride. (From Wharen RE, Anderson RE, Laws ER: Quantitation of hematoporphyrin derivative in human gliomas, experimental central nervous system tumors, and normal tissues. *Neurosurgery* 1983: 12:446–450. Used by permission.)

TABLE 13–1.
Concentration of HPD in Experimental Tumors*

TUMOR	HISTOLOGY	TIME AFTER INJECTION, HR	FLUORESCENCE, μG/ML	HPD, μG/GM
1	Glioma	24	1.3	1.0
2	Neurinoma	24	0.9	0.5
3	Neurinoma	24	1.1	1.5
4	Neurinoma	4	18	...
5	Spinal cord ependymoma	4	0.25	0.30
6	Neurinoma	4	11	10.7
7	Spinal cord ependymoma	4	13	10.9
8	Neurinoma	4	11	10.2

* HPD indicates hematoporphyrin derivative. Tumors were induced by ethylnitrosourea. Concentrations of HPD were measured after the intraperitoneal injection of 10 mg/kg.

TABLE 13–2.
HPD Concentration in Biopsy Specimens From Patients During PRT*

DIAGNOSIS	HPD, μG/GM TISSUE	TIME FOLLOWING HPD ADMINISTRATION, HR
Grade 3 L frontal oligodendroglioma	0.1	48
Grade 3 L parietal astrocytoma	2.5	24
Grade 3 R frontal astrocytoma	1.7	24
Cerebellar medulloblastoma	10	6
Fourth ventricle ependymoma	6	6

* HPD indicates hematoporphyrin derivative; PRT, photoradiation therapy.

to 0.1 μg/gm 24 hours after HPD administration, wherease at 4 hours there was approximately 0.3 μg/gm. It is interesting that in one case of a spinal-cord ependymoma, very little HPD was observed, similar to what Rasmussen-Taxdal et al. observed in 1955.[39] Thus, although HPD does concentrate in tumor tissue, HPD is not completely excluded by the blood-brain barrier, as a small amount of HPD is present in the normal brain during PRT. Whether or not this small amount of HPD can be damaging to the normal brain is an important question currently under investigation. Experimentally, predominantly in rats, there is no doubt that under the appropriate conditions there is some toxicity to normal brain.[3,6,40] Clinically, however, within the parameters that have been used in our clinical trials, this has not been a problem. It appears that the parameters of PRT can be adjusted to limit the toxicity to normal brain, but further studies in this regard are needed.

Using this microfluorescence assay, HPD has been quantitated in a series of biopsy specimens from patients during PRT (Table 13–2). The HPD concentration 24 hours following the intravenous administration of 5 mg/kg of HPD was approximately 1 μg/gm, whereas at 4 hours it was 10 μg/gm. Surrounding brain tissue yielded values of 0.1 to 0.3 μg/gm at 4 hours and 0.1 μg/gm 24 hours following HPD administration. These values are similar to the results obtained with experimental tumors and give some indication of the HPD concentration achieved in human brain tumors.

Investigations of the parameters of HPD photocytotoxicity of human glioma cells in cell culture have been performed using a trypan blue exclusion assay (Fig 13–3).[1,46,48] The action spectrum of human glioma cell HPD photocytotoxicity corresponds with the absorption spectrum of HPD and is consistent with reports of action spectra of different human cell lines.[1,27,35]

Cell survival curves following violet and red light irradiation at a power density of 20 mW/sq cm demonstrated a consistent pattern with an increasing slope and decreasing shoulder to the curve and increasing concentrations of HPD. The cellular killing efficiency varied linearly with HPD concentration. The relative killing efficiency of violet light compared with red light irradiation was approx-

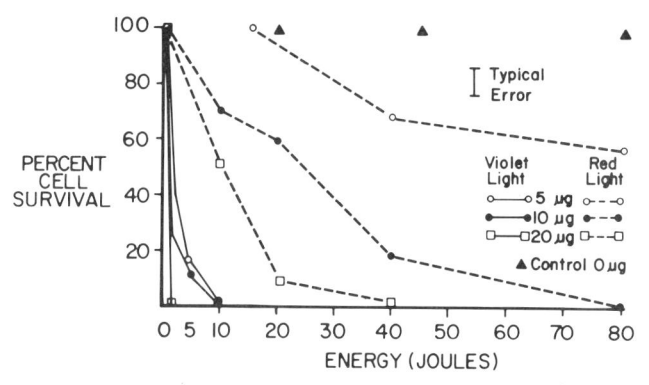

FIG 13-3.
Survival curves of U87MG human glioblastoma cells following irradiation with violet (400 nm) and red (630 nm) light at a power density of 20 mW/sq cm. Before irradiation, the cells were exposed to hematoporphyrin derivative at concentrations of 0, 5, 10, and 20 µg/ml for 24 hours. Typical error represents the SD of three independent determinations for each survival curve. (From Wharen RE, So S, Anderson RE, et al: Hematoporphyrin derivative photocytotoxicity of human glioblastoma in cell culture. *Neurosurgery* 1986; 19:495–501. Used by permission.)

imately 12:1, which coincides with previous studies[1,27] and reflects the relatively poor absorption of HPD for red light. Red light is used in PRT, however, because it provides maximal tissue penetration of visible light through normal brain by approximately 1,000-fold compared with violet light.[38]

As discussed previously, quantitation of the amount of HPD in biopsy specimens of gliomas from patients 24 hours following the intravenous administration of 5 mg/kg of HPD revealed levels of 1 to 10 µg/ml. Human glioma cells exposed to 1 and 10 µg/ml of HPD for 24 hours in cell culture required 25 and 100 J of red light, respectively, at a power density of 20 mW/sq cm to achieve 50% cell killing, and 80 J was required at 10 µg/ml HPD for 100% cell killing. Since there is no difference in the killing efficiency at power densities from 10 to 100 mW/sq cm for red light,[1] this suggests that at least 80 J/sq cm of red light exposure would be necessary effectively to kill glioma cells during PRT at power densities of 10 to 100 mW/sq cm. As the HPD concentration decreases, even greater energies would be required to achieve cytotoxicity. Although Cheng et al.[6] have demonstrated that power densities below 50 mW/sq cm produced no significant hyperthermic response in normal rat brain, whether this magnitude of light exposure presents any significant toxicity to normal brain at similar HPD concentrations is unknown. Initial clinical studies[29,34] might suggest that such energy levels are well tolerated, but further, carefully controlled investigation is necessary.

Spikes demonstrated in 1975 that porphyrin sensitized photo-oxidations involved the production of an excited triplet state of the dye that can react with biologic substrates either directly (type I photo-oxygenation) through the production of free radicals or indirectly (type II photo-oxygenation) through the production of singlet molecular oxygen.[41,42] Dougherty proposed in 1976[14] that singlet oxygen was the cytotoxic agent for the in vitro inactivation of TA3 mouse mammary carcinoma cells exposed to HPD photoirradiation using red light. Further work has demonstrated that, although most porphyrin-sensitized reactions occur via a type II mechanism involving singlet oxygen,[41,44,45] other type I mechanisms may be important under certain conditions.[11,22,25]

The effect of oxygen concentration on HPD phototoxicity of human glioma cells (Fig 13–4) reveals that cellular killing efficiency increased directly with increasing Po_2 values from 12 to 490 mm Ha using red light at a density of 100 mW/sq cm. The enhancement of cellular killing efficiency by increased oxygen availability to the cell was approximately fivefold between 84 and 490 mm Hg. However, at very low Po_2 values, below 12 mm Hg, there was a slight but consistent increase in killing efficiency that was not due simply to a cellular hypoxia, as the survival of control cells was 100% at a Po_2 of 7 mm Hg.

The direct relationship between cytotoxicity and Po_2 from 12 to 490 mm Hg suggests that reactive oxygen species are involved in the phototoxic process and that HPD photocytotoxicity of human glioma cells can be enhanced by increasing the oxygen availability to the cell. Cytotoxicity does occur, however, even at low oxygen concentrations. Lee et al.[30] have suggested that the oxygen present in the system can be reused to generate the toxic species because prolonged irradiation at low oxygen concentration can increase phototoxicity to an extent approaching the cytotoxicity achieved under atmospheric conditions.

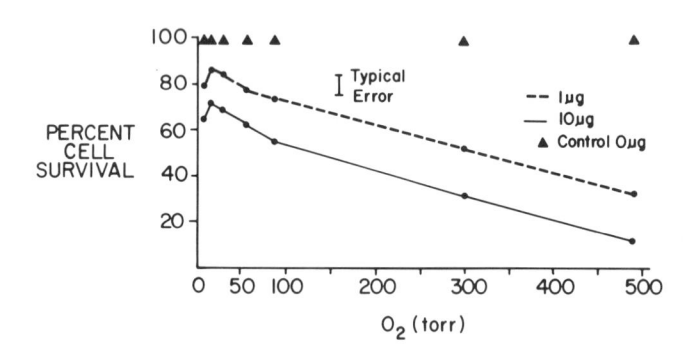

FIG 13–4.
Survival curves of U87MG human glioblastoma cells at oxygen tensions (O_2) of 7 to 490 mm Hg (torr) following irradiation with 40 J of red light (630 nm) at a power density of 100 mW/sq cm. Before irradiation, the cells were exposed to hematoporphyrin derivative at concentrations of 1 and 10 µg/ml for 24 hours. (From Wharen RE, So S, Anderson RE, et al: Hematoporphyrin derivative, photocytotoxicity of human glioblastoma in cell culture. *Neurosurgery* 1986; 19:495–501. Used by permission.)

Further studies[48] have demonstrated that HPD phototoxicity can be effectively quenched by β-carotene, an effective quencher of singlet oxygen. This quenching effect of β-carotene is most evident at the higher Po_2 values. Mannitol, a quencher of free hydroxyl ion radicals, however, had no effect on the cellular killing efficiency for Po_2 values from 30 to 490 mm Hg. This supports the hypothesis that the preferred mechanism of the cytotoxic effect of HPD is by singlet oxygen and not free radical formation. However, the consistent increase in cytotoxicity at Po_2 values less than 12 mm Hg suggests that at very low Po_2, cytotoxicity may occur through other mechanisms. Indeed, Foote[18] has stated that the relative efficiency of type I and type II reactions depends on the various concentrations of oxygen substates and triplet sensitizer as well as the rate constant for each reaction and the rate for the spontaneous decay of the excited triplet state. Apparently at very low Po_2 values, cytotoxicity either began to occur via mechanisms other than singlet oxygen or the cell for some reason became more sensitive to singlet oxygen destruction. Regardless of the mechanism, however, it is apparent that HPD photocytotoxicity of human glioma cells can be effective even under hypoxic conditions.

After all the drug and light parameters have been maximized in HPD PRT, the limiting factor in its clinical application may remain the penetration of light through brain and tumor tissue.[13,46] Svaasand et al.[43] have demonstrated that the penetration depth, which is the distance in which red light is attenuated by 90% in adult brain, is on the order of 1.5 mm. If that is the case, then the depth of penetration of light at 630 nm represents a significant limitation for the use of PRT in brain tumors. It is known, however, that the penetration of light through tissue continues to improve by several orders of magnitude as the wavelength increases from 600 μm to 1.1 nm.[38] Thus, the possibility exists that PRT at these wavelengths might provide a more effective depth of penetration.

CLINICAL STUDIES

In parallel with the laboratory investigations, clinical experience has expanded slowly but steadily. The majority of patients have had recurrent malignant gliomas, and prior attempts at therapy had failed. Photoradiation therapy has thus far been applied by two methods. Initial attempts involved the stereotaxic insertion of a fiberoptic probed into deep-seated lesions delivering red light (630 nm) produced by an argon-pumped dye laser. More recently, HPD PRT has been applied by irradiating the tumor bed with filtered light from a xenon arc lamp following resection of the tumor, both for recurrent tumors and occasionally at the time of the initial resection.

Hematoporphyrin derivative is usually administered (following sterile preparation) as a piggyback infusion at a dose of 3 to 5 mg/kg over 5 to 10 minutes into a freely running intravenous line of D_5 0.2% normal saline. Thus far, there has been no toxicity associated with the administration of HPD in this manner.

Thirty-one patients have received HPD PRT. The initial six patients had deep-seated lesions treated with dye pumped argon laser by stereotaxic insertion of a quartz fiber, whereas the other 25 patients have received xenon arc lamp (red light) irradiation of the tumor bed following resection. Initially, patients received PRT approximately 24 hours after administration of the drug, but after the laboratory studies suggested that higher tumor levels of HPD were achieved at a shorter time interval, PRT has been applied approximately 6 hours after HPD administration. In seven patients, a light diffusion medium was used by filling the cavity of the tumor bed with the medium to disperse the light evenly across the tumor bed.

The majority of the patients treated by HPD PRT (Table 13–3) have involved recurrent tumors, predominantly gliomas. There have been three cases of metastasis and five cases involving posterior fossa tumors. In two cases (one medulloblastoma and one ependymoma), PRT was administered at the time of the initial resection. The case of a craniopharyngioma was a multiply recurrent cystic tumor in which HPD was placed stereotaxically into the cyst. After 15 minutes, a quartz fiber was stereotaxically placed into the cyst and PRT administered.

Figure 13–5 is an example of one of the early cases. The patient was a 75-year-old right-handed man with a grade 4 left frontal astrocytoma initially treated by resection and radiation therapy. The computed tomographic (CT) scan in Fig 13–5,A is a recurrence 5 months following the initial surgery. He subsequently received PRT through a quartz fiber using 400 mW/sq cm of red light (630 nm) from an argon pumped laser for 40 minutes. A CT scan performed one month after PRT treatment (Fig 13–5,B) reveals only a slight decrease in the size of the lesion. He subsequently died 8 months following PRT and 13 months after his initial resection.

Figure 13–6 demonstrates another early case, of a 14-year-old right-handed girl with a grade 3 left thalamic astrocytoma initially biopsied and subtotally resected in 1980. She subsequently received 5,500 rad of radiation therapy. In December 1980, she was treated with PRT via a quartz fiber (300 mW/sq cm

TABLE 13–3.
HPD PRT of Brain Tumors*

PATHOLOGY	NO. OF CASES
Glioma	21
Metastasis	3
Ependymoma	3
Medulloblastoma	2
Craniopharyngioma	1
Rhabdomyosarcoma	1

* HPD indicates hematoporphyrin derivative; PRT, photoradiation therapy.

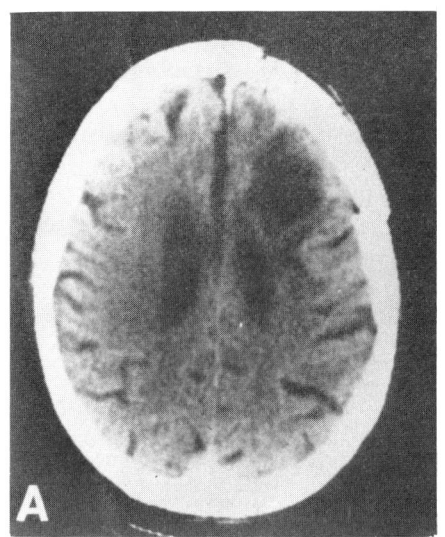

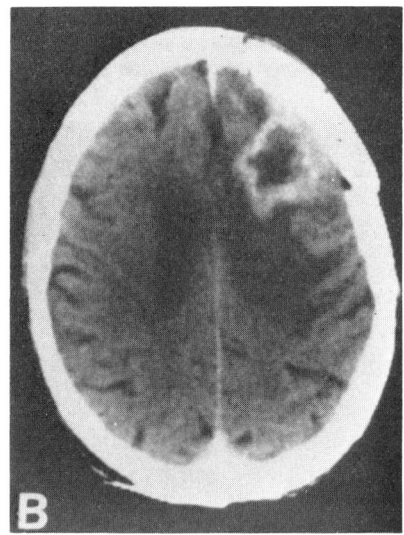

FIG 13–5.
Left frontal grade 4 astrocytoma before (**A**) and 1 month after (**B**) photoradiation therapy. (From Laws ER, Cortese DA, Kinsey JH, et al: Photoradiation therapy in the treatment of malignant brain tumors: A phase I (feasibility) study. *Neurosurgery* 1981; 9:672–678. Used by permission.)

for 60 minutes). She tolerated the procedure well and was discharged one day after her treatment. Her postoperative scan demonstrates only a slight decrease in the size of the lesion. However, although she has had the cystic portion of the tumor drained on one other occasion, her most recent CT scan in January 1986, is essentially unchanged.

Results of the six early cases of patients treated with interstitial PRT for recurrent malignant gliomas (Table 13–4) reveals a median survival of approximately 10 months following HPD PRT. There have certainly been no cures, and whether the therapy has been of benefit to these patients is difficult to know. These cases do demonstrate, however, both the feasibility of the technique and the fact that the technique is capable of tumor cell destruction. It now appears that the major problem with this technique is the limited penetration of light through brain tissue,[13,46] and because of this HPD PRT has little if any potential for killing off large volumes of tumor.

Because HPD PRT is effective in killing glioma cells but limited by the ability of light to penetrate tissue, we thought that the technique could be applied most effectively by delivering the PRT to the tumor bed after resection of the tumor. In this situation, we hope the remaining tumor cells would be within the depth of light penetration. Twenty-five patients have now received PRT administration to the tumor bed following resection of the tumor, 16 of whom had recurrent malignant gliomas. Results thus far in these 16 patients reveal a mean survival of 11 months for the eight patients who have died. Two patients are alive with recurrence and the longest survival without recurrence is four years. All have received red light at 50 to 100 mW/sq cm for 30 to 60 minutes from a filtered xenon arc lamp. Our results with malignant gliomas are similar to those reported by McCulloch et al.,[34] who found that patients with gross total removal of their

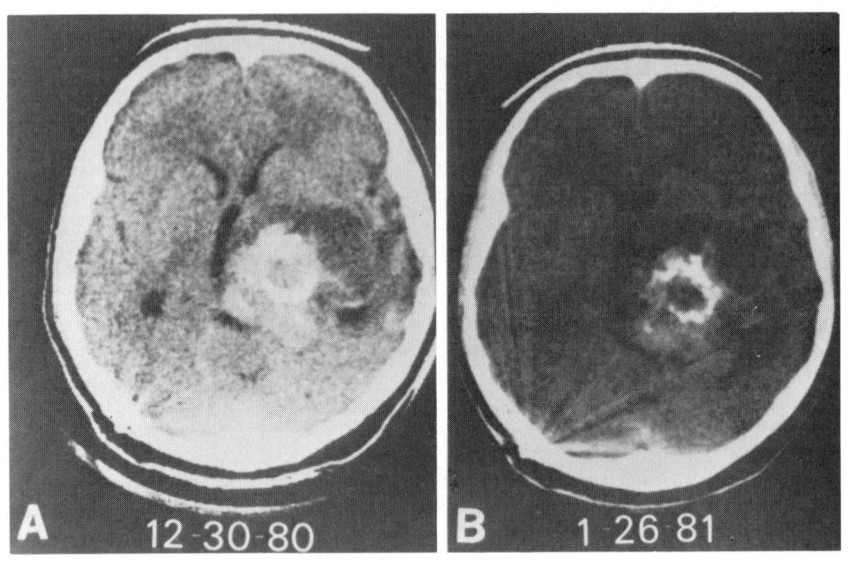

FIG 13–6.
Left thalamic grade 3 astrocytoma before (**A**) and 1 month after (**B**) photoradiation therapy. (From Laws ER, Cortese DA, Kinsey JH, et al: Photoradiation therapy in the treatment of malignant brain tumors: A phase I (feasibility) study. *Neurosurgery* 9:672–678. Used by permission.)

TABLE 13–4.
Results of Interstitial HPD PRT of Recurrent Gliomas*

		630-NM LASER TECHNIQUE		
PATIENT NO.	PATHOLOGY	DENSITY, mW/SQ CM	DURATION, MIN	RESULTS
1	Grade 3 R frontal astrocytoma	300	30	Alive, 15 mo
2	Grade 4 L frontal	400	60	Dead, 5 mo
3	Grade 3 L temporal	325	45	Dead, 4 yr
4	Grade 3 R frontal astrocytoma	400	60	Dead, 4 mo
5	Grade 4 R frontal astrocytoma	250	30	Alive, 19 mo

* HPD indicates hematoporphyrin derivative; PRT, photoradiation therapy.

TABLE 13-5.
HPD PRT of Posterior Fossa Lesions*

		POSTRESECTION XENON ARC TECHNIQUE			
PATIENT NO.	PATHOLOGY	WAVELENGTH, NM	DENSITY, mW/SQ CM	DURATION, MIN	RESULTS
1	Medulloblastoma	White	100	30	Alive, 40 mo
2	Medulloblastoma (recurrent)	620	50	30	Alive, 22 mo
3	Ependymoma	630	100	20	Alive, 6 mo
4	Ependymoma	630	50	40	Alive, 17 mo
5	Ependymoma	405	10	40	Died, DIC

* HPD indicates hematoporphyrin derivative; PRT, photoradiation therapy; DIC, disseminated intravascular coagulation. In patients 2 and 4 a diffusion medium was used.

TABLE 13-6.
HPD PRT of Metastatic Lesions*

		POSTRESECTION TECHNIQUE		
PATIENT NO.	PATHOLOGY	DENSITY, mW/SQ CM	DURATION, MIN	RESULT
1	L parietal adenocarcinoma (lung)	20	60	Alive with recurrence, 20 mo
2	L frontal melanoma	10	60	Alive, 18 mo
3	R frontal adenocarcinoma (colon)	100	30	Alive, 6 mo

* HPD indicates hematoporphyrin derivative; PRT, photoradiation therapy. Xenon arc laser (630 nm) was used. In patients 1 and 2 a diffusion medium was used.

tumors followed by PRT of the tumor bed had the best results. However, in contrast to the patients described by McCulloch et al. with malignant gliomas, none of our patients has received PRT at the time of the initial resection.

The most encouraging cases thus far have involved the application of PRT to the tumor bed following gross total resections of posterior fossa tumors (Table 13-5). In two cases (one medulloblastoma and one ependymoma), PRT was applied at the time of the initial resection. The 10-year-old boy with medulloblastoma is now alive without recurrence at 40 months. One patient died of disseminated intravascular coagulation. Otherwise, in this group in which PRT was administered to the region of the fourth ventricle and brain stem, there have been no complications.

Three patients with metastatic tumors have received HPD PRT (Table 13-6) and thus far have done well. Two are alive without recurrence at 6 and 18 months, whereas the third is alive with recurrence at 30 months following treatment.

The patient with the multiply recurrent left-orbit rhabdomyosarcoma in an enucleated globe was treated early in our series and died two months after therapy.

In this case, PRT was applied at 12, 24, and 36 hours after HPD administration, and at each treatment approximately a centimeter of tumor sloughed. Unfortunately, the patient with the multiply recurrent cystic craniopharyngioma who received PRT stereotaxically into the cyst died 4 months following the treatment from a pulmonary embolus.

Overall, the technical aspects of these clinical trials in patients with brain tumor have been quite satisfactory and the treatment well tolerated. There have been no adverse effects related to the administration of HPD. Complications have included two wound infections, both of which responded to antibiotics, and two cases of cutaneous photosensitivity in patients who disregarded advice to protect themselves from direct sunlight. Using power densities of less than 200 mW/sq cm of red light, cerebral edema has not been a problem. All of our patients received steroids before and after treatment. Only one patient in our series developed prolonged postoperative edema either from the surgical resection or from the PRT. The two deaths have been discussed previously.

Our conclusions thus far regarding the application of HPD PRT for brain tumors are as follows: (1) the technique can effectively and selectively kill tumor cells and can be safely applied to patients; (2) the potential of HPD PRT is limited by the penetration of visible light through brain tissue; (3) the technique is incapable of eradicating large volumes of tumor; and (4) the technique may be applicable as an adjunctive treatment in selected cases although no conclusions can be made thus far regarding its efficacy. The results, however, are encouraging for several reasons. The theoretical basis of PRT is sound, and the treatment is well tolerated and practical to use. Finally, at least some of the patients appear to have derived some benefit.

We hope that as the basic knowledge of PRT and malignant brain tumors increases and further laboratory work in cell cultures and in animal systems progresses, it will be possible to improve the efficiency and efficacy of PRT. Clinical indications may expand as well to include the treatment of nonmalignant but invasive brain tumors such as meningiomas, pituitary adenomas, and craniopharyngiomas. The combination of PRT with other methods, such as stereotaxic carbon dioxide laser resection, hyperthermia, or radiation, may ultimately help to achieve control of these devastating tumors. Finally, HPD is certainly not an ideal photosensitizer, and the search continues for more effective drug-light combinations, particularly at longer wavelengths with a greater ability to penetrate brain tissue. Recent reports[28] have suggested that HPD can be activated by conventional radiation and that HPD may be an effective radiosensitizer. If this turns out to be the case, then the problem of tissue penetration might be solved, which might change the approach of PRT entirely.

ACKNOWLEDGMENTS

We are grateful to Peggy Apel and Dr. Garth Powis, Department of Oncology Research, Mayo Clinic, for their assistance with the cell cultures, and to Jill Nicklas for her assistance in preparing the manuscript.

REFERENCES

1. Anderson RE, Wharen RE, Jones CA, et al: Parameters of hematoporphyrin derivative tumor cell killing efficiency: Decomposition of hematoporphyrin derivative at high power densities, in Doiron DR, Gomer CJ (eds): *Porphyrin Localization and Treatment of Tumors.* New York, Alan R Liss, 1983, pp 483–500.
2. Benson RC, Farrow GM, Kinsey JH: Detection and localization of in situ carcinoma of the bladder with hematoporphyrin derivative. *Mayo Clin Proc* 1982; 57:548–555.
3. Berenbaum MC, Hall GW, Hoyes AP: Cerebral photosensitization by hematoporphyrin derivative: Evidence for an endothelial site of action. *Br J Cancer* 1986; 53:81–89.
4. Bodaness S, Chan PC: Singlet oxygen as a mediator in the hematoporphyrin catalyzed photooxidation of NADPH+ to NADP+ in deuterium oxide. *J Biol Chem* 1977; 252:8554–8560.
5. Carpenter RJ III, Neel HB III, Ryan RJ, et al: Tumor fluorescence with hematoporphyrin derivative. *Ann Otol Rhinol Laryngol* 1977; 86:661–666.
6. Cheng MK, McKean J, Boisvert D, et al: Effects of photoradiation therapy on normal rat brain. *Neurosurgery* 1984; 15:804–810.
7. Cheng MK, McKean J, Mielke B, et al: Photoradiation therapy of 9L-gliosarcoma in rats: Hematoporphyrin derivative (types I and II) followed by laser energy. *J Neurooncol* 1985; 3:217–288.
8. Cortese DA, Kinsey JH: Hematoporphyrin derivative phototherapy for local treatment of cancer of the tracheobronchial tree. *Ann Otol Rhinol Laryngol* 1982; 91:652–655.
9. Dahlman A, Wile AG, Berns MW: Laser photoradiation therapy of cancer. *Cancer Res* 1983; 43:430–434.
10. Diamond, I, Granelli SG, McDonagh AF, et al: Photodynamic therapy of malignant tumors. *Lancet* 1972; 2:1175–1177.
11. Dixit R, Mulchtarh, Bickers DR: Destruction of microsound cytochrome P-450 by reactive oxygen species generated during photosensitization of hematoporphyrin derivative. *Photochem Photobiol* 1983; 37:173–176.
12. Doiron DR (ed): *The Clayton Foundation Symposium on Porphyrin Localization and Treatment of Tumors.* New York, Alan R Liss, 1983, pp 24–28.
13. Doiron DR, Svaasand CO, Profio AE: Light dosimetry in tissue application to photoradiation therapy. *Adv Exp Med Biol* 1981; 160:63–76.
14. Dougherty TJ: Photodynamic therapy (PDT) of malignant tumors. *CRC Crit Rev Oncol Hematol* 1984; 2:83–116.
15. Dougherty TJ, Dridey GB, Fiel R, et al: Photoradiation therapy: II. Cure of animal tumors with hematoporphyrin and light. *JNCI* 1975; 55:115–119.
16. Dougherty TJ, Kaufman JE, Goldfarb A, et al: Photoradiation therapy for the treatment of malignant tumors. *Cancer Res* 1978; 38:2628–2635.
17. Dougherty TJ, Lawrence G, Kaufman JH, et al: Photoradiation therapy in the treatment of recurrent breast carcinoma. *JNCI* 1979; 62:231–237.
18. Foote CS: Mechanisms of photosensitized oxidations. *Science* 1969; 162:963–970.

19. Foote CS: Mechanisms of photoxygenation; in Doiron DR, Gomer CJ (eds): *Porphyrin Localization and Treatment of Tumors.* New York, Alan R Liss, 1984, pp 3–18.
20. Forbes IJ, Cowled PA, Leong AS, et al: Phototherapy of human tumors using hematoporphyrin derivative. *Med J Aust* 1980; 2:489–493.
21. Granelli SG, Diamond I, McDonagh AF, et al: Photochemotherapy of glioma cells by visible light and hematoporphyrin. *Cancer Res* 1975; 35:2567–2570.
22. Grossweiner CI, Patel AS, Grossweiner JB: Type I and type II mechanisms in the photosensitized lysis of phosphatidylcholine liposomes by hematoporphyrin. *Photochem Photobiol* 1982; 36:159–167.
23. Hyata Y, Kato H, Konaka C: Hematoporphyrin derivative and laser photoradiation in the treatment of lung cancer. *Chest* 1982; 81:269–277.
24. Hisazumi H, Misaki T, Miyoshi N: Photoradiation therapy of bladder tumors. *J Urol* 1983; 130:685–687.
25. Jori G, Reddi E, Tomio L, et al: Factors governing the mechanism and efficiency of porphyrin-sensitized photoxidations in homogenous solutions and organized media, in Kessel D, Dougherty TJ (eds): *Porphyrin Photosensitization.* New York, Plenum Publishing Corp, 1983, pp 193–212.
26. Kelly J, Snell ME, Berenbaum MC: Photodynamic destruction of human bladder carcinoma. *Br J Cancer* 1975; 31:237.
27. Kinsey JH, Cortese DA, Moses HL, et al: Photodynamic effect of hematoporphyrin derivative as a function of optical spectrum and incident energy density. *Cancer Res* 1981; 41:5020–5026.
28. Kostron H, Swartz MR, Miller DC, et al: The interaction of hematoporphyrin derivative, light, and ionizing radiation in a rat glioma model. *Cancer* 1986; 57:964–970.
29. Laws ER, Cortese DA, Kinsey JH, et al: Photoradiation therapy in the treatment of malignant brain tumors: A phase I (feasibility) study. *Neurosurgery* 1981; 9:672–678.
30. Lee See K, Forbes W, Betts WH: Oxygen dependency of photocytotoxicity with hematoporphyrin derivative. *Photochem Photobiol* 1984; 39:631–634.
31. Lipson RL, Baldes EJ: The photodynamic properties of a particular hematoporphyrin derivative. *Arch Dermatol* 1960; 82:508–516.
32. Lipson RL, Baldes EJ: Photosensitivity and heat. *Arch Dermatol* 1960; 82:517–520.
33. Lipson RL, Baldes EJ, Olsen AM: The use of a derivative of hematoporphyrin in tumor detection. *JNCI* 1961; 26:1–8.
34. McCulloch GA, Forbes IJ, Lee See K, et al: Phototherapy in malignant brain tumors; in Doiron DR, Gomer CJ (eds): *Porphyrin Localization and Treatment of Tumors.* New York, Alan R Liss, 1984, pp 709–718.
35. Moan J, Christiansen T, Jacobsen PB: Porphyrin-sensitized photoirradiation of cells in vitro, in Dorion DR, Gomer CJ (eds): *Porphyrin Localization and Treatment of Tumors.* New York, Alan R Liss, 1984, pp 419–442.
36. Perria C, Capuzzo T, Cavagnaro G: First attempts at the photodynamic treatment of human gliomas. *J. Neurosurg Sci* 1980; 24:119–129.
37. Perria C: Photodynamic therapy of human gliomas by hematoporphyrin and He-Ne laser. *IRCS Med Sci Cancer* 1981; 9:57–58.
38. Preass LE, Bolin FP, Cain BW: Tissue as a medium for laser light transport implications for photoradiation therapy, in Goldman L (ed): *Lasers in Medicine and Surgery. Proc SPIE* 1982; 357:77–84.

39. Rassmussen-Taxdal DS, Ward GE, Figge FJH: Fluorescence of human lymphatic and cancer tissue following high doses of intravenous hematoporphyrin. *Cancer* 1955; 8:78–81.
40. Rounds DE, Jacques S, Shelden CH: Development of a protocol for photoradiation therapy of malignant brain tumors: I. Photosensitization of normal brain tissue with hematoporphyrin derivative. *Neurosurgery* 1982; 11:500–505.
41. Spikes SD: Porphyrins and related compounds as photodynamic sensitizers. *Ann NY Acad Sci* 1975; 244:496–508.
42. Spikes SD: Photobiology of porphyrins, in Doiron DR, Gomer CJ (eds): *Porphyrin Localization and Treatment of Tumors*. New York, Alan R Liss, 1984, pp 19–40.
43. Svaasand CO, Ellingsen R: Optical properties of human brain. *Photochem Photobiol* 1983; 38:293–299.
44. Tse PT: Photoradiation therapy in the management of intraocular, orbital, and periocular tumors. Read before the First International Conference on the Clinical Applications of Photosensitization for Diagnosis and Treatment, Tokyo, April 30 to May 2, 1986.
45. Wharen RE, Anderson RE, Laws ER: Quantitation of hematoporphyrin derivative in human gliomas, experimental central nervous system tumors, and normal tissue. *Neurosurgery* 1983; 12:446–450.
46. Wharen RE, Anderson RE, Laws ER: Photoradiation therapy with hematoporphyrin derivative in the management of brain tumors, in Fasano VA (ed): *Advanced Intraoperative Technologies in Neurosurgery*. New York, Springer Verlag, 1986, pp 211–227.
47. Wharen RE, Anderson RE, Laws ER: Laboratory and clinical investigations of HpD photoradiation therapy of malignant brain tumors: Technique and results in 31 patients. Read before the First International Conference on the Clinical Applications of Photosensitization for Diagnosis and Treatment, Tokyo, April 30 to May 2, 1986.
48. Wharen RE, So S, Anderson RE, et al: Hematoporphyrin derivative (HpD) photocytotoxicity of human glioblastoma in cell culture. *Neurosurgery* 1986; 19:495–501.
49. Wile AG, Dahlman A, Burns MW: Laser photoradiation therapy of recurrent human breast cancer and cancer of the head and neck, in Kessel D, and Dougherty TJ (eds): *Porphyrin Photosensitization*. New York, Plenum Publishing Corp, 1983, pp 47–52.
50. Wile AG, Novatry J, Mason GR, et al: Photoradiation therapy of head and neck cancer. *Am J Clin Oncol* 1984; 6:39–43.
51. Wise BL, Taxdal DR: Studies of the blood-brain barrier utilizing hematoporphyrin. *Brain Res* 1967; 4:387–389.

Index

A

Ablation, 113, 129
  excimer laser and, 16
  vascular surgery and, 114
Absorption, 25, 129
Absorption spectrum, 138
Accreditation Manual for Hospitals, 31
Acridine orange dye, 137
Aerodigestive tract, 6
Air filter, 34
Aluminum tape, 36-37
American Congress of Laser Neurosurgery, 7
American National Standards Institute, 27
Anastomosis, 3
  carbon dioxide laser and, 15
  laser-assisted microvascular, 112
  laser at site of, 111
Anesthesia
  general, 46
    with neuromuscular blockade, 42
    upper airway surgery and, 36-37
  local, 46
  regional, 46
Anesthesiologic considerations, 40-48
  brain surface in, 41-46
  neuroanesthesia in, 46-47
  personnel and patient safety in, 40-41
Aneurysm, 8
  obliteration of, 133
  surgical application for, 113
Angioblastoma, 106
Angiography, 91
Anterior cervical procedure, 40
Anterolateral cordotomy, 124
Anterolateral meningioma, 102
Apneic oxygenation, 43
Arachnoidal plane, 49
Argon gas, 14
Argon-ion laser, 3, 8, 13, 21
  aneurysm obliteration and, 133

  anterolateral cordotomy and, 124
  commissural myelotomy and, 124
  DREZ lesion and, 124
  intradural tumor and, 106
  laser-tissue interaction and, 129
  ophthalmology and, 14
  pediatric neurosurgery and, 60
  petrous tumor and, 56, 57
  photocoagulation and, 14
  retina and, 14
  safety and, 28, 35, 40
  structure of, 14
  theoretical neurosurgery and, 129-136
Argon-pumped dye laser, 163
Arterial pulsation, 42
Arterial pulse pressure, 44, 45
Arteriovenous malformations, 113
Articulated arms, 23
Ascher, Peter W., 6
Astrocytoma, 77, 103
  frontal, 164
  pilocytic, 96-97
  thalamic, 164
Avalanche breakdown, 22
AVMs (*see* Arteriovenous malformations)
Avulsion, cervical root, 125

B

Basal ganglia tumor, 93
Beck, Oskar J., 8
Beta-carotene, 163
Biliary stone, 16
Biochemical cellular changes, 110
Biolaser technician, 38
Biologic tissue transparency, 143
Biopigments, 142-143
Bipolar electrical technique, 114
Bleeding ulcer, 21
Blood
  flow of, 25

loss of, 60
optical density of, 143
Blood-brain barrier, hematoporphyrin derivative and, 141
Blood pressure reduction, 47
Boggan, J., 8
Bottle neurinoma, 103
Brain
   extra-axial tumor of, 49
   lesions of, 61-66
   management of, 40
   surface, 41-46
   motion of, 41, 42
   pulsation of, 45
   systemic effect of lesioning of, 132
Brain glioma operation, 6
Brain tumor (see Malignant brain tumors)
Breast, carcinoma of, 100
Brillouin scattering, 22
Bureau of Radiological Health, 27
Burn debridement, 4

C

Capsule of tumor
   entry point of, 50
   irradiation of, 50
   shrinkage of
      intracapsular, 50-51
      petrous tumor and, 56
Capsulotomy, 21
Carbon dioxide laser, 1, 2, 3-7
   advantage of, 15
   anastomosis and, 15
   anterolateral cordotomy and, 124
   beam delivery for, 23-24
   brain lesions and, 61-66
   coefficient of absorption of, 105
   commissural myelotomy and, 124
   deep tumor and, 92
   DREZ lesion and, 124, 132
   dumb-bell neurofibroma and, 101
   electrical hazard and, 33
   gliomas and, 49
   hemostatic properties of, 5
   intradural tumor and, 106
   intraspinal meningioma and, 102
   laser-tissue interaction and, 129
   maintenance and, 34
   medial sphenoid lesion and, 53
   meningiomas and, 49
   nerve welding and, 134
   neuroablation and, 115
   pediatric neurosurgery and, 60
   petrous tumor and, 56, 57
   reparative technique, 114
   safety and, 28, 33-34, 40
   smoke evacuation and, 35-36
   structure of, 15
   syringohydromyelia and, 116
   theoretical neurosurgery and, 129-136
   third-degree burns and, 28
   tumor removal and, 104
   vaporization of, 49-50
   vascular application and, 110-114
Carbon dioxide laser microslad, 93
Carbonization, 131
Carcinoma, 100, 101
Cardiovascular diseases, 21-22
β-Carotene, 163
Cavitation, cystic spinal cord, 115
Cell changes, 110, 143
Cerebellopontine angle tumor, 55
Cerebral edema, 148
Cerebral vascular resistance, 44
Cerullo, Leonard, 7
Cervical decompression, 74
Cervical procedures, anterior, 40
Cervical root avulsion, 125
Chalcogenide glass, 24
Chemotherapy, 98
Chiari I malformation, 118
Chiari II deformity, 73-76
Children
   blood loss in, 60
   fenestration in, 77
   nervous system of, 60
Chromophores, 25
Clivus tumor, 54-55
Coagulation, 8
   deep-vessel, 15
   as effect of laser, 104
Coagulation necrosis, 131
Commissural myelotomy, 124-125
Congenital anomalies, 61
Congenital lesion, 66
Contralateral motor weakness, 132
Convexity tumor, 52
Cooling system of carbon dioxide laser, 34

INDEX

Cordotomy, 124
Cranial vault, 42
Craniopharyngioma, 167
Craniotomy
   extra-axial tumor removal and, 49
   stereotaxically guided, 90
   trephine, 90, 95
Credentialing of nurses and physicians, 31-33
CT/MRI-compatible stereotaxic head frame, 90
CT scanning, 96, 116
Cystic spinal cord cavitation, 115

D

DA (*see* Digital angiography, stereotaxic)
Deafferentation pain, 125
Debulking, 56
Decompression, 74
Decompressive laminectomy, 100
Deep tumor, 93-97
Deep-vessel coagulation, 15
Dermal sinuses, 70-72
Dermoid tumor, 70-72
Descarte's law, 19-20
Devascularization of tumor pedicle, 51
DHE (*see* Dihematoporphyrin ether)
Diastematomyelia, 72
Diatomic molecules, 15
Dielectric waveguide scalpel, 22
Digital angiography, stereotaxic, 91
Dihematoporphyrin ether, 138
DNA, excimer laser and, 16
Dorsal root entry zone lesion, 125, 132-133
Dosimetry, light, 142-145
DREZ lesion (*see* Dorsal root entry zone lesion)
Drying of tissue, 110
Dumb-bell neurinoma, 102-103
Dumb-bell neurofibroma, 101
Dura
   neurinoma within, 102
   tissue welding and, 134
Dye, acridine orange, 137
Dye laser, 16

E

Edema
   cerebral, 148
   of white matter, 92
   zone of, 131
Educational criteria, 32
Edwards, M.S.B., 8
Electrical hazard, 33
Electric methods of monitoring, 46
Electromagnetic radiation, 10
Endoscopy, 18
Endotracheal tube, 36
Energy and depth of lesion, 130
Ependymoma, 103
   photoradiation therapy and, 167
Epicerebral microcirculation, 131
Epidermoid tumor, 106
Epidural carcinoma, metastatic, 100, 101
Epidural tumor, 77, 100
Equilibrium temperature, 145
Equipment malfunction, 31
Excimer laser, 21
   structure of, 15-16
Exposure time, 110, 112
External beam radiation therapy, 98
Extinction length, 129
Extra-axial tumor
   removal of, 49-59
      clivus tumor and, 54-55
      convexity tumor and, 52
      foramen magnum tumor and, 55
      lateral sphenoid tumor and, 52
      medial sphenoid lesion, 52-54
      petrous tumor and, 55-58
      planum sphenoidale tumor and, 54
      steps in, 51
   surgical approach to, 58
   vaporization of, 49
Extradural tumor, 100-101, 106
Extramedullary tumor, 77
E-YAG laser, 16-17
Eye, 15

F

Fasano, A., 8
FDA, 27
Federal safety regulation, 29-30
FEL laser, 17-18
Fenestration, 117
   in children, 77
Fiberoptic probe, 163

Fidler, James, 4
Filter, air, 34
Filum terminale, 68
Fire, 40-41
Fluoride glass, 24
Foramen magnum tumor, 55
Fox, J.L., 8
Frank-Starling relationship, 45
Frontal astrocytoma, 164
Frontal lobe, 86-87
Fusion, healing after, 111

G

Gas supply, 34
Gastrointestinal tract tumor, 100
General anesthesia, 46
  with neuromuscular blockade, 42
Glial neoplasm (*see also* Gliomas)
  biologic characteristics of, 83-84
  conventional and stereotactic applications in, 82-99
    biologic characteristics and, 83-84
    goals and, 84-85
    laser and, 85-86
    surgical approaches and, 86-98
Glioblastomas, 6
Gliomas (*see also* Glial neoplasm)
  carbon dioxide laser and, 49
  photoradiation and, 163, 165
  surgery and, 98
    brain, 6
    goals in, 84-85
    surgical laser in, 85-86
Goldman, Leon, 4
Gold vapor laser, 16
Gynecologic microsurgery, 6

H

Halogen atoms, 15
Head frame, stereotaxic, 90
Healing after fusion, 111
Heat dissipation, 18
Hemangioma, 106
Hematoporphyrin, 137
  brain tumors and, 156
  complications from use of, 168
  malignant gliomas and, 163-164
  photocytotoxicity parameters of, 160, 162, 164
Hematoporphyrin derivative, 137-155, 138
  blood-brain barrier and, 141
  dye laser and, 16
  malignant brain tumor and, 147
  photochemotherapy with
    cerebral edema and, 148
    complication of, 148
    hyperthermic effect and, 145
Hemoglobin, 25
Hemostasis, 8, 50, 87
  carbon dioxide laser and, 4-5
  intramedullary tumor and, 103
HeNe laser, 35
Heppner, F., 6
HF laser, 16-17
Histologic changes, 131-132
HPD (*see* Hematoporphyrin derivative)
Hydromyelia, 76
Hyperthermia, phototherapy and, 145
Hypertonic solution, 143
Hypocapnia, 45
Hypophysectomy, 126
Hypotonicity, 143

I

Industrial Hygienists, 27
Infant, blood loss in, 60
Injury from laser, 27
Intracapsular tumor, 50-51
Intracranial glioma surgery, 86-97
  centrally located superficial lesions and, 90-92
  deep tumor and, 93-97
  polar lesion and, 86-90
Intracranial pressure, 132
Intradural tumor, 106-107
  extramedullary, 77, 101-103
Intramedullary tumor, 68, 77, 103-105, 116
Intraspinal chordoma, 106
Intraspinal meningioma, 102
Intraspinal tumor, 100-109
  extradural tumor, 100-101
  intradural-extramedullary tumor, 101-103
  intramedullary, 103-105

Intraspinal tumor (*cont.*)
  unusual, 106-107
Iophendylate, 116, 118
Ischemia, spinal cord, 72

J

Jain, K.K., 8
Jako, Geza J., 5
Joint Commission on Accreditation of Hospitals, 27

K

Kiefhaber, Peter, 7
KRS-5 (*see* Polycrystalline thallium bromoiodide)
Krypton laser, 28, 35

L

L (*see* Extinction length)
Laminectomy
  decompressive, 100, 101
  extra-axial tumor removal and, 49
  syringohydromyelia and, 116
Laryngeal microsurgery, 6
Laser
  advantages of, 5
  argon-ion (*see* Argon-ion laser)
  argon-pumped, 163
  carbon dioxide (*see* Carbon dioxide laser)
  classification of, 30
  components of, 13
  definition of, 10
  delivery of, to tumor, 144
  development of, 10-26
  dye, 16
  E-YAG, 16-17
  excimer, 15-16, 21
  FEL, 17-18
  generation of, 11-13
  gold vapor, 16
  HeNe, 35
  HF, 16-17
  history of, 10-26
  krypton, 28, 35
  mode-locked, 12
  neodymium:YAG (*see* Neodymium:YAG laser)
  principles of, 10-26
  role of, 1-9
  structure of, 10-26
  thermal effect of, 130
  thermal energy of, 105
  tissue effect and, 24-25
  types of, 13-18
  visible and near-infrared, 20-23
Laser fiber-balloon irradiator, 144, 145
Laser fiber tips, 144
Laser lesion, 130, 131
Laser safety officer, 38-39
Laser safety technician, 38
Laser syringostomy, 112
Laser-tissue interaction, 129
Lasing medium, 13
Lateral sphenoid tumor, 52
Law, 31
Lawsuit, 31
Lesion
  brain, 61-66
  congenital, 66
  depth of, energy and, 130
  dorsal root entry zone, 125, 132-133
  high-grade, 97
  laser, 130, 131
  low-grade, 97
  medial sphenoid, 52-54
  recurring, 98
  size of, 130
  spinal, 66-79
  superficial, 90-92
Liability, preceptor, 31
Light
  biopigments and, 142
  optical fibers and, 20-23
Light dosimetry, 142-145
Light fluency, 145
Lipoma
  of filum terminale, 68
  intramedullary, 68
  spinal cord, 67, 68
Lipomeningocele, 67-70
Lobectomy, frontal, 86-87
Local anesthesia, 46
Logarithmic relation of energy and lesion depth, 130
Lung carcinoma, 100

M

Maiman, T.H., 1, 13
Maira, G., 8
Malignant brain tumors
  hematoporphyrin derivative and, 147
  photoradiation of, 147, 156-171
    clinical studies in, 163-168
    laboratory investigations in, 158-163
    red light and, 147
Malignant gliomas, 163, 165
Medial sphenoid lesion, 52-54
Medical device law, 30
Medulloblastoma, 167
Melanin, 25
Meningioma, 6, 101
  anterolateral, 102
  carbon dioxide laser and, 49
  intraspinal, 102
  olfactory-groove, 156
  of petrous bone, 55
  subdural, 102
Meridional rays, 19
Metastatic carcinoma, 100, 101
Metrizamide myelography, 116
Meyer-Schwickerath, G., 1
Microcirculation, 131
Microfluorescence assay, 159
Micromanipulator, 7
Microslad, carbon dioxide laser, 93
Microsurgery
  gynecologic, 6
  intramedullary tumor and, 103
  laryngeal, 6
Microvascular anastomosis, 112
Mode-locked laser, 12
Molecules, diatomic, 15
Morcellation, intracapsular, 50-51
Motor weakness, contralateral, 132
MRI imaging, 96, 116
Mutagenesis, 16
Myelocystocele, 72
Myelomeningocele, 72, 73
Myelotomy, commissural, 124-125
Mylar tape, 37

N

Nath, Gunther, 7
ND:YAG laser (*see* Neodymium:YAG laser)
Nd-in-glass laser, 7
Necrosis, coagulation, 131
Neodymium laser, 2
Neodymium:YAG laser, 1, 7-8, 21 (*see also* YAG laser)
  bloody neoplasm and, 57
  laser-tissue interaction and, 129
  pediatric neurosurgery and, 60
  petrous tumor and, 57
  safety and, 28, 34, 40
  structure of, 14-15
  theoretical neurosurgery and, 129-136
  third-degree burns and, 28
  tissue welding and, 133
Neoplasm, 61-66 (*see also* Glial neoplasm; Tumor)
  bloody, 57
  intramedullary, 77
  malignant, 156, 157 (*see also* Malignant brain tumors)
  pain due to, 122
  in pediatric spinal disease, 66-67
  spinal cord, 77-78
  surgical modulation of intractable pain and, 115
Nerves
  anastomoses and, 134
  tissue welding and, 134
Nerve tumor, acoustic, 55
Nervous system of children, 60
Neural tissue, 129-132
Neurectomy, 126, 133
Neurinoma, 101, 133
  bottle, 103
  dumb bell, 102-103
  within dura, 102
Neuroablation, 115-128
  carbon dioxide laser and, 115
  pain and, 122-126
  syringohydromyelia and, 115-122
Neuroanesthesia, 46-47
Neurofibroma, 101
Neurogenic pain, 125
Neuroma (*see* Neurinoma)
Neuromicrosurgery, 7
Neuromuscular blockade, 41, 42
Neurosurgery
  anesthesia management and, 40
  history of, 1-9

Neurosurgery (cont.)
  monitoring and, 46
  pediatric, 60-81
  photoradiation therapy and, 158
  stereotaxic laser and, 95
  theoretical, 129-136
    laser sources and, 129-132
    specific applications, 132-133
    tissue welding, 133-134
Nitrogen carbon dioxide laser, 3-4
Norton tube, 37
Nurses
  certification of, 32-33
  clinical laser, 37-38
  credentialing of, 31-33

O

Occipital lobectomy, 89-90
Occupational Safety and Health Administration, 27
  regulations of, 30
Olfactory-groove meningioma, 156
Operating microscope, 6
Operating room conduct, 40
Ophthalmology, argon-ion laser and, 14, 35
Optical density of blood, 143
Optical fibers, 24
  light propagation and, 20-23
  principles of, 19-20
Organic tissue
  fusion potential of, 111
  reconstruction of, 111-113
Oxygen, hematoporphyrin phototoxicity and, 162
Oxygenation, apneic, 43

P

Pain, 122-126
Pantopaque (see Iophendylate)
Paraplegia, traumatic, 125
Patel, 2
Patient care, 40
Patient safety, 40-41
PCT (see Photochemotherapy)
PDT (see Photodynamic therapy)
Pediatric neurosurgery, 60-81
  brain lesions in, 61-66

spine lesions in, 66-79 (see also Spinal lesions)
Pedicle of tumor, devascularization of, 51
Penetrance distance, 142
Periventricular tumor, 93
Personnel safety, 40-41
Petrous tumor, 55-58
Photoactivation spectrum, 138
Photochemical reaction, 16
Photochemotherapeutic activity, 143
Photochemotherapy, 137-155
  cerebral edema and, 148
  clinical experience and, 147-148
  complication of, 148
  hematoporphyrin derivative with, 147-148
  light dosimetry and, 142-145
    total dose of light delivered in, 143
  malignant brain tumor and, 147
  photosensitizer and, 138-142
  thermal consideration and, 145-147
Photocoagulation, argon-ion laser and, 14
Photocytotoxicity of hematoporphyrin, 160, 162, 164
Photodynamic therapy, 16, 137
Photo-oxidation process, type II, 139
Photophysical parameter of sensitizer, 137
Photoradiation therapy, 98
  malignant brain tumors and, 156-171
    clinical studies in, 163-168
    laboratory investigations in, 158-163
  neurosurgery and, 158
Photosensitizer, 137, 138-142
  absorption spectrum of, 138
  properties of, 156
Phototoxicity of hematoporphyrin, 160, 162, 164
Physicians, credentialing of, 31-33
Pilocytic astrocytomas, 96-97
Planum sphenoidale tumor, 54
Plasma shock wave, 25
Polar lesion, 86-90
Polycrystalline fiber, 24
Polycrystalline thallium bromoiodide, 23-24
Polyvinyl chloride endotracheal tube, 36
Population inversion, 10
Porphyrins, 137
Port wine stain, 16

Posterior fossa decompression, 74
Posterior fossa tumors, 167
Preceptor's liability, 31
Proprioceptive impairment, 125
Prostatic carcinoma, 100
Protein as absorber, 25
Pulse, factors producing, 44
Pulse pressure reduction, 45
Pyryliums, 149

Q

Q-switching, 12

R

Radiation, electromagnetic, 10
Radiation therapy
 external beam, 98
 metastatic cord compression and, 100
Radiofrequency generator, 125
Radiofrequency techniques, 132
Raman scattering, 22
Reconstructed effect, 111-113
Red light, brain tumors and, 157
Refractive index, 19
Regional anesthesia, 46
Renin-angiotensin system, 132
Reparative effect, 113-114
Retinal bleeding, 14
Retinal reattachment, 14
Retractor, stereotaxic surgical, 94
RF generator (see Radiofrequency generator)
RF techniques (see Radiofrequency techniques)
Rhizotomy, 126
Ruby laser, 1
 pulsed, 2
 safety and, 40

S

Safety
 laser, 27-39
 personnel and patient, 40-41
Sealing response, 113
Self-focusing, 22
Sensitizer, photophysical parameter of, 137

Shrinking response, 113
Sinuses, dermal, 70-72
Skin sensitivity to sunlight, 148
Skull base procedure, 40
Smoke evacuation, 35-36
Somatosensory evoked potentials, 116, 117
Spatial modes, 13
Spectrum, absorption, 138
Sphenoid lesions, 52-54
Spinal arachnoiditis, 116
Spinal cord (see also Spinal lesions)
 cystic cavitation of, 115
 extra-axial tumor of, 49
 intramedullary tumor of, 116
 surgical removal of, 105
 motion of, 41
 safety and, 40, 41-46
 surface management of, 41-46
 trauma to, 116
Spinal disease, pediatric, 66-79 (see also Spinal lesions)
Spinal dorsal root entry zone lesions, 132
Spinal lesions, 66-79, 100-109 (see also Spinal cord)
 Chiari II deformity in, 73-76, 77, 78, 79
 dermal sinuses in, 70-72
 dermoid tumors in, 70-72
 extradural, 100-101, 106
 intradural-extramedullary, 101-103, 106-107
 intramedullary, 103-105
 lipomas in, 67-70
 lipomeningocele in, 67-70
 myelomeningocele in, 73
 spinal cord neoplasms in, 77-78
 syringohydromyelia in, 76-77
 tethered cord in, 72-73
Spinothalamic tract, 124
Spot size, 112
Steam formation, 131
Stellar, 5
Stereotaxic digital angiography, 91
Stereotaxic frame, 93
Stereotaxic laser neurosurgery, 95
Stereotaxic serial biopsy, 98
Sterotaxic surgical retractor, 94
Stereotaxically guided craniotomy, 90
Stoke's photon, 22

Index

Strong, M. S., 6
Structural-cellular changes, 110
Subcortical lesion, extirpation of central, 90
Subdural lipoma, 106
Subdural meningioma, 102
Sunlight, skin sensitivity to, 148
Surgical field, movement of, 41
Surgical retractor, stereotaxic, 94
Syringohydromyelia, 76-77, 115-122
    structural abnormality of, 115
    treatment modalities for, 116
Syringostomy, laser, 112
Systemic vascular resistance, 44

T

Tape, aluminum, 36-37
Teflon, 24
Teleradiographs, anteroposterior and lateral, 96
Temperature
    changes of, 130-131
    exposure time and, 110, 112
    of laser-irradiated tissue, 25, 105, 130-131
    low levels of, 110
    photochemotherapy and, 145-147
Temporal lobe, 87-89
Temporal lobectomy, 87-89
Teratoma, epidermoid, 106
Tethered cord, 72-73
Thalamic tumor
    hematoporphyrin and, 164
    stereotaxic laser approach to, 93
Thermal effect
    exposure time and, 110
    of laser, 25, 105, 130-131
    of photochemotherapy, 145-147
Thermal energy of laser light, 105
Thermal scale, applications of, 110-114
Third-degree burns, 28
Thyroid carcinoma, 100
Time, exposure, 110, 112
Tissue
    ablation of, 129
    drying of, 110
    laser-irradiated, temperature of (*see* Temperature)
Tissue effect of laser, 24-25

Tissue welding, 133-134
Todd Wells stereotaxic frame, 92
Toxic combustion, 40-41
Toxicity of hematoporphyrin, 160, 162, 164
Tracheostomy, 36
Transmandibular approach to foramen magnum tumor, 55
Transoral approach to foramen magnum tumor, 55
Transparency of biologic tissue, 143
Transsphenoidal procedure, safety and, 40
Transverse gaussian profile, 22
Traumatic paraplegia, 125
Trephine craniotomy, 90, 95
Tumor (*see also* Spinal lesions)
    basal ganglia, 93
    carbon dioxide laser in removal of, 104
    in cerebellopontine angle, 55
    clivus, 54-55
    convexity, 52
    deep, 93-97
    dermoid, 70-72
    devascularization of pedicle of, 51
    epidermoid, 106
    epidural, 77, 100
    extra-axial (*see* Extra-axial tumor)
    extradural, 100-101, 106
    extramedullary, 77
    of foramen magnum, 55
    of gastrointestinal tract, 100
    intradural-extramedullary, 101-103
    intramedullary, 68, 77, 103-105, 116
    intraspinal (*see* Spinal lesions)
    lateral sphenoid, 52
    malignant brain, 156-171 (*see also* Malignant brain tumors)
    morcellate chunk of, 50
    movement of, during surgery, 95
    planum sphenoidale, 54

U

Ulcer, bleeding, 21
Ultrasonography, 116
Undulator, 17, 18

Upper airway surgery, anesthesia safety during, 36-37
Urinary stones, 16
Uterus, 21

V

Vaporization
  area of, 131
  intracapsular, 50-51
Vascular application of thermal scale, 110-114
Vascular lesions of brain, 61
Vascular pedicle, 51
Vascular resistance, 44
Ventilation, 42
  high-frequency, 43
  shallow, 43
Ventilatory motion, 42
  apneic oxygenation and, 43
Vessels, 44
  brain lesion and, 61
  thermal scale and, 110-114
  tissue welding and, 133-134
  tumor pedicle and, 51
von Hippel-Lindau disease, 106

W

Water as absorber, 25
Waveguide mode, 20
Welding, tissue, 133-134
Whispering-gallery waveguide, 23
White matter, tumor cells in, 92
Wyburn-Mason disease, 106

X

Xenon arc lamp, 143
Xenon light, 35

Y

YAG laser (*see also* Neodymium:YAG laser)
  intradural tumor and, 106
  petrous tumor and, 56, 57
  sphenoid lesion and, 52, 53
Yttrium aluminum garnet, 14 (*see also* YAG laser)

Z

Zirconium fluoride, 24

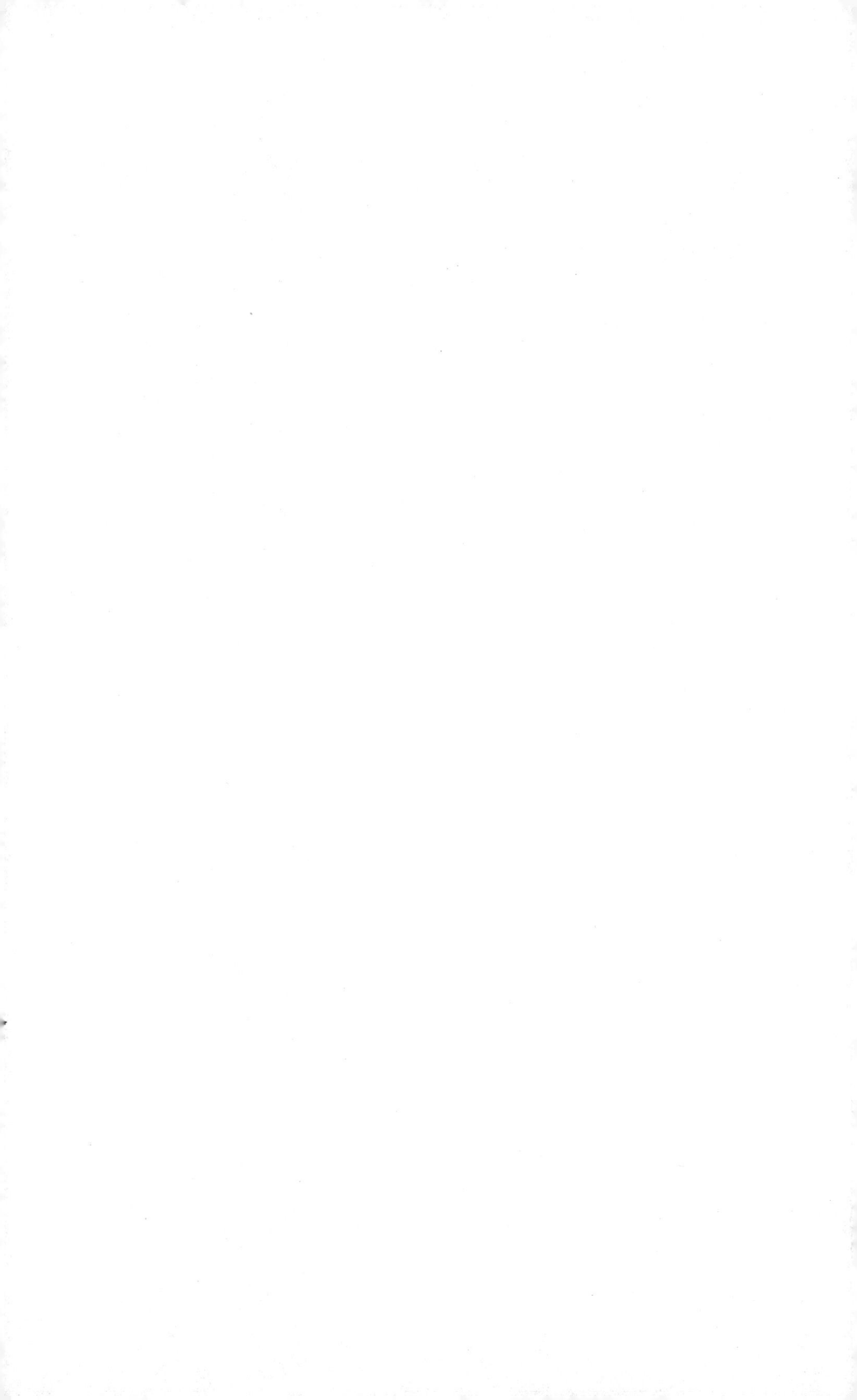